CONVERSION DISORDER

CONVERSION DISORDER

LISTENING TO THE BODY
IN PSYCHOANALYSIS

JAMIESON WEBSTER

Columbia University Press
New York

Columbia University Press
Publishers Since 1893
New York   Chichester, West Sussex
cup.columbia.edu
Copyright © 2019 Columbia University Press
Paperback edition, 2022
All rights reserved

Library of Congress Cataloging-in-Publication Data
Names: Webster, Jamieson, author.
Title: Conversion disorder : listening to the body
in psychoanalysis / Jamieson Webster.
Description: New York : Columbia University Press, [2018] |
Includes bibliographical references and index.
Identifiers: LCCN 2018016929 (print) | LCCN 2018037283 (ebook) |
ISBN 9780231184083 (cloth) | ISBN 9780231184090 (pbk.) |
ISBN 9780231545310 (e-book)
Subjects: LCSH: Conversion disorder. | Psychoanalysis.
Classification: LCC RC532 (ebook) | LCC RC532 .W425 2018 (print) |
DDC 616.89/17—dc23
LC record available at https://lccn.loc.gov/2018016929

Cover design: Lisa Hamm
Cover image: © plainpicture / Uwe Reicherter

FOR SIMON CRITCHLEY

CONTENTS

INTRODUCTION 1

I. DAYBREAK 29

II. MUSIC OF THE FUTURE 61

III. FATHER CAN'T YOU SEE 87

IV. NEVER THE RIGHT MAN 101

V. I AM NOT A MUSE 117

VI. HYSTERICAL RUINOLOGY 135

VII. *COITUS INTERRUPTUS* 155

VIII. THREE VISIONS OF PSYCHOANALYSIS 179

IX. HOW TO SPLINTER / HOW TO BURN 203

X. FORGED IN STONES 215

XI. THE SLIDING OF THE RING 237

XII. THE ANALYST'S ANALYSIS 253

Acknowledgments 273

Appendix 275

Notes 283

References 291

Index 297

INTRODUCTION

Who has the courage for psychoanalysis anymore? Or, to put it another way, who has the time and the energy in a world where "being busy" is one's raison d'être? Forty-five minutes, three or four or even five times a week—with the terror that this arrangement will last a decade, maybe longer, two. Even before all of this, one has to find an analyst, always first a stranger, resulting in an arrangement whose peculiar contours are not only longer than most of today's marriages but require more concentrated time, more investment in disruption, futility, vulnerability, repetition, and the desire for radical change, without even the slightest guarantee or indication of what's to come. Maybe we should ask: How much suffering is necessary before one turns to psychoanalysis, when one can see an endless string of medical doctors, body healers, psychics, or coaches or rely on the habitual comfort of friends and family? What must fail in the response of these others to suffering that makes the psychoanalyst necessary?

Who has the courage to be a psychoanalyst in a world uninterested in the kind of change, idealistic or not, that psychoanalysis offers? Who has the courage to take on this unbalanced task, which promises the perpetuation of pain more than its alleviation? Who has the courage to lend little more than an ear in a world gone deaf—deaf despite hypercommunication and information overload? What can the analyst ask of a patient when the patient is to do the asking?

Patients come to you with a history of insufficient health care, several attempts via Eastern medicine to fend off the heavy hands of surgical and pharmacological intervention, and feeling the responsibility for their unease squarely on their shoulders alone. The responsibility is theirs, despite how obvious it is—the salt in the wound—that society has failed them in so many ways. This sense of responsibility almost immediately transforms into guilt (even when the manifest affect is outrage), a guilt shorn of the tenderness that religion can offer and caught instead in an ethos of personal consumerism that hides more in homes and phones than in any space held in common. The patient—who wants to be an educated patient, a wise consumer—meets the psychoanalyst amid a relentless fear of being duped and at a moment when they are desperate to find help, to find someone to unburden themselves to and with. None of this can be a lament for the psychoanalyst or a place to lodge nostalgia. Freud wanted us to enter into a common human unhappiness, into a sober sense of what is possible. Sometimes I want to kick him. Who has the courage for that?

When a patient comes, what does the psychoanalyst ask? Typically, I ask patients to speak and to tell me their dreams. When I say this to patients, who are undoubtedly excited on some level by the prospect, I feel ridiculous. Am I some kind of obscurantist, an anachronism, whose point of reference is a century back, too long ago for anyone even to remember enough to despise it in the timelessness of the present? "Obsolete" isn't even a good enough word to describe how silly this can sound when others have *things* to give—pills and worksheets and evidence and advice. Even with a sense of the esteemed place that dreams have held in religion and literature and history, patients can see me as nothing more than a voyeur, playing out this game of nighttime talk for my own intellectual curiosity. "Clearly you like dreams, but what does that have to do with me?"

This general refusal to provide proof, pills, promises, or polish is taken as a sign either of my impotence or, on the other end, of pure sadism—I'm never really certain of which until the patient lashes out. Yes, these attitudes that surround the psychoanalyst would already be a workable transference of some kind, that is, if they weren't so universal, soldered to a therapeutic worldview that deemed psychoanalysis wrong a long time ago. For transference to function as part of the treatment, it has to rest on something more specific and unique in the patient's history. It is not simply a warm bath of negativity that mirrors a general sentiment. The initial demand for help, simultaneous with an extensive skepticism toward analysts and their methods, is not part of the treatment in the same way that a specific resistance in an already functioning transference would be. What kind of space can there be in first meetings between incredulous strangers? How can a treatment even begin this way?

General wisdom states that resistance is best dealt with through submitting to the patient, by continuing to listen as generously as possible, hoping that this allows the patient to drop their guard or at least decide if they want to. Yes, why are you here asking for help from something as ridiculous as a psychoanalyst? If the treatment carries on, the psychoanalyst can gently refuse everything but the painful exchange of literal nonsense from the evening ephemera of dreams, the stutters of the attempt simply to speak—especially about sex—and the vague outlines of a history of suffering—especially at the hands of others. If one is a classical psychoanalyst, one doesn't interpret much—asking questions, working with patients slowly, taking these dreams apart, listening for the logic that has determined the life of their symptoms. One can do this without giving anything that resembles concrete meaning or advice.

The interpretation will come on its own account; this takes time, maybe even years. One cannot underestimate the reign of misrecognition. This kind of work in psychoanalysis, little by little, begins to chart a path, developing a rhythm that gives the treatment a definitive shape—what Freud would call its architecture. For anyone who has witnessed this slow transformation—the force of this work to create the subtlest yet most radical shifts—there isn't room for a lot of doubt, except perhaps concerning how to find the way to break into this space with every patient. On the shoulders of the analysts lies the majority of the responsibility for this possibility without, however, the promise that it will be possible. Who has the patience, let alone the courage?

ANXIETY

One of the conundrums I find myself in is that the clinical picture doesn't seem to have changed much at all, meaning that the direction of the work is framed in a manner more or less concordant with what I have learned from Freud. At the same time, the diagnostic nomenclature has mushroomed in a peculiar vacuum, available to all as a part of public discourse. The psychiatric manual is statistically defined and controlled, a closed logical system—yet it is simply a model of the consensus attained by a rarified group of ever-changing psychiatrists and clinicians, evident enough in the fact that the classifications change drastically and chaotically from one edition to another. They follow fads or reject them, incorporating them into a system that takes in the demands of the day.

This is not an either/or—my old Freudian model or today's psychiatric categories. Rather, what today's system shows me is its porous relation with the world, its force as a system that can exist on the outside, while psychoanalysis preserves itself, hidden in a kind of fold, away from the flux of the contemporary landscape. I'd like to oblige the structural model, closed in one sense, also to take on the changing climate, not to change with it—which is what current psychiatry does—but to open itself up in a way that it can meet what is outside.[1] This might begin to show us the margin of responsibility for preserving the old while forcing it into contact with the present.

None of this—this question of clinical diagnosis, the outlines of contemporary mental health—needs to matter in the strong scientific sense, determining what is true. Take, for example, the mere fact that patients now read about their diagnoses, usually on the internet, often because they are curious about those strange numbers that appear on their therapy bills, all of which gives the system a life of its own, one increasingly independent from its makers. The seduction of finding oneself on the outside touches something specific in each patient and grabs hold of them. What is this meeting point? My wager, founded in an unfounded idolatry of Freud, is that this meeting of inside and outside is precisely what is magnificent about how he worked—and also, that it is rare. We tend toward the extremes of open and closed rather than the interplay and rhythm of their difference. The psychoanalyst, the discourse about the psychoanalyst—set against medicine, philosophy, religion, psychiatry, psychology, self-help, and so on—is already implicated in the unconscious.

We can scour the web, search endless chat groups whose sole purpose is to identify heartily with a supposed disorder. Whether you choose to identify with any such community, the bonds and the language forged are there to be "witnessed" by all. The choice seems to be whether you take the poison alone or among others, giving a certain shape to an identification with being sick. I say this without wishing in the slightest to return to some point in history when psychiatric knowledge belonged only to psychiatrists, like the Bible reserved for the few who spoke Latin. It isn't as if religion saved us from identifying with illness. What I want to indicate instead is something singular about the present moment and the value of the anachronism of being a psychoanalyst. We may have lost recognition, but that does not mean we do not have a place, especially in a world that embraces the idea of being "mentally ill," whatever that might mean.

A patient comes to you complaining of anxiety. They have read everything on the internet about anxiety disorders and the meditation or mindfulness techniques for abating it. They've researched benzodiazepines and probably have tried their friend's prescription. They've gone through the rounds of herbalists, body workers, stress massage, breathing techniques, cleanses, and journaling. They've even cut out gluten. But what they are seeking in all this is something more. The desire to place terribly real and painful bodily feelings somewhere grows more and more intense. Is my illness caused by biology or circumstance or ancestry? They'll often settle for all three, being better equal opportunists than the mental-health ideologues. To what in this panacea does the psychoanalyst respond?

After having listened carefully, usually less to the efficacy of their attempts to cure themselves and more for the temporal sequence in the irruption of symptoms, I tell them they can do what they like, that some of these things are helpful, but that the only way I can deal with their anxiety is not to talk about it but to try and talk. Imagine! The problem is that I understand anxiety structurally, that is, as a difficulty in relation to separation, especially separation from anxiety. Often a patient's anxiety manifests as a demand for the analyst to deny separation and become overinvolved with him or her. Communication, according to Lacan, is predicated and haunted by the denial of separation.

Anxiety has always been one of the greatest threats to the psychic system in Freud, who continued to refine his theory of anxiety till the end of his life. Anxiety isn't merely a negative force; rather, it is a question of a mass, a quantity to which we must form a relationship. It demands palpable change in a system. Separation is part of the work of analysis. It is structural, taking place at the border between inside and outside, something you can do miraculously simply by speaking. It takes time. Separation is not something you have achieved or not; rather, anxiety speaks loudly about a separation that is never simply there. Anxiety concerns the liminal aspects of subjectivity, including something in sexuality that highlights separateness and makes bearing it difficult. Anxious patients love their anxiety and stick close to it, monitor it, greet it like a long-lost friend, especially the kind of friend we keep in order to complain about.

We also happen to live in a time that is deeply invested in the vicissitudes of anxiety, a time of deep insecurity, of paranoia and too much communication, too many nonchoices. Though we have a thousand palliative techniques at our disposal, we are in a closed, almost claustrophobic loop. This loop mirrors the problem of being trapped by anxiety—an anxiety that, in fact, has no outside. This is why it tends toward either claustrophobia, on the one hand, or agoraphobia, on the other. I take this cultural read incredibly seriously, and I believe the diagnosis is right. We live in a time of high anxiety, and we are facing the breakdown of collective fantasy. Nevertheless, anxiety and the work of separation have always been necessary, even if the latter is more necessary than ever.

Freud said that most cures follow the lines of mass psychology or collective fantasy in the guise of religion or philosophies of life. They bind anxiety in a collective illusion that covers over the fact of separation. One might even say that collective anxieties *are* our new religion—giving way to all kinds of new rituals, from meditation apps to social media.

Psychoanalysis wants to reintroduce a separation that always fails to take place; this is one way of characterizing neurosis, creating new solutions to the fundamental anxieties of living that aren't simply one more "crooked cure."[2]

Patients with anxiety suffer from what seems like an excess of interiority. This leaves them vulnerable to the repeated fantasy of controlling the outside world, as if such mastery might help them enter into it, help them separate from the anxiety that takes them over from the inside. The problem seems less a lack of "proper" interiority or interior equilibrium (whatever that would be) but actually that there may be no "real" outside or no way into this "outside." Patients come concerned about parts of their external reality—money, family, love, work, physical pain—which they think and think and think about without pause, and the thoughts become more and more empty. The problem is that neither a defined inside nor outside exists either in the vagaries of anxiety or in collective resistances. What can arrive on the scene as a differentiating edge? What conversion of this energetic stasis can be found?

If psychoanalysis has lost its way, perhaps we need to return to the question of how we understand any supposed inside or outside—or, to put it another way, how psychoanalysis creates change. This is certainly part of what is at stake in this book on conversion disorder: conversion in the sense of radical reinvention and the aptitude, as Freud called it, for transposing large quantities of excitation, a process that has the effect of restructuring one's psyche. To transpose something from one place to another creates a cut, a separation. Conversion requires an intimacy with the ordeal of psychoanalysis: what it disorders and reorders and how these disorders meet with the disorder of the world. Above all, why analysts cannot be made anxious by their patients easily. This is the problem with the hysterical contagion of anxiety.

Why would this be a breaking point—for me, for psychoanalysis, or for patients (and their many attempts to cure themselves)? I think that it takes more courage than ever to continue the work of psychoanalysis. To continue without the energy of invention and newness. Without the security of professional authority. While psychoanalysis flourishes under conditions of impossibility—which is why what I write here is not simply a complaint and is perhaps more a call to order—one has to recognize, at the very least, what we are up against. Again, who has the courage?

CURE

Many analysts talk of the joys of the work, the intimacy with patients, the pleasure of watching them fulfill their potential, and so on. This is true, yet I think these serve as palliative gestures and essentially false promises. The work is difficult and uncertain, and the pressures are greater than ever. There is an assault on the authority of the analyst even as we are still defining what it means to be "cured"—leaving many new therapists uneasy when they have yet to finish their own analyses. I wouldn't easily qualify anything as pleasurable, especially being a psychoanalyst. As far as I'm concerned, all pleasure comes from the unconscious, and it takes time to know this—in oneself, to say nothing of for another—and to tolerate what is ephemeral about a pleasure that is besieged when it isn't barred. When patients finally access more pleasure in their life, the analyst is often the last to know.

The cliché that the analyst will remember more of the treatment than the patient, for whom so much of it disappears behind the veil once a treatment ends, lends itself to the idea that the work is special. This gesture can be dangerous. I think we like to tell ourselves that the work is so wonderfully rewarding because we face this radical erasure. Something about the absolute nature of a patient's leaving treatment has always been present in the literature on termination, speaking to how the patient's intense investment in the analyst's presence is completely overturned in a sudden process of mourning and separation. One doesn't know what happens to patients—that is, except in the case of one's own analysis, oneself as a patient. Analysts are in the unique position to know something about the continued life of their own analysis, how it lives on in their work as analysts, while also being the sole repository for the memory of so many analyses. Is the burden of knowledge part of the impossibility? Being the only one to have to hold all of this?

Responsibility, personal or professional, requires a relationship to the unknown that demands care. What have we done or not done? Perhaps psychoanalysis highlights something extreme in responsibility. So much of the hand-wringing about the profession is directed at this impossibility—tell us what you are going to do, prove the effect you will have! We proceed in the dark, yet the many renditions of psychoanalysis often obscure this fact, promising this, that, and the next thing in some analytic afterlife. This promise was Freud's main diagnosis of religious salvation as a response to an infantile wish. I'm not here to denounce the confusion of psychoanalysis with the wish for salvation. We could look at how this wishing is passed down, how it erupts in an analysis, and how it finds a point of resolution. We could ask what the wish for conversion has to do with neurotic myths of salvation and what psychoanalysis changes differently for a patient. What in a psychoanalytic conversion would be distinctly different from what religion sutures?

The courage for this impossible profession is supposed to come from the analyst's own analysis—a practice that many have rightly called psychoanalysis's pyramid scheme. It is—but, on the other hand, this work demands a huge sacrifice to accommodate these would-be analysts in an analysis that must go further than any other—that must do something more than make a patient's life more livable. I don't think psychoanalysis "saves" you, at least not for those who become analysts. Perhaps this is the "more"—this particular shattering of what is in excess of the question of livable life. On the other side, for the analyst, the pressures of training analyses (as they are now called) are so unbelievably great: the intensity of the transference and the demand on the side of the trainee-patient, whose identification with his or her analyst is both an iatrogenic inevitability and the greatest obstacle in a treatment's success.

No one can understand the kind of scrutiny training analysts face until they are on the other side—this fact has engendered some of the most bitter professional wars in psychoanalysis, centered on the question of who can psychoanalyze these would-be-analysts. How this situation breaks in one direction or another is the lynchpin of the field's survival, something that every analyst must be held responsible for. This is an added burden when what termination is remains the largest blind spot in the profession, which points to the poverty of relevant literature on the topic but also to what in the question must remain indeterminate.

The necessity to find a way through this pressure is infinite. It is interminable. In Freud's famous last paper on the question of termination, we might understand this word—"*Unendliche*"—as speaking more to the analyst than the patient. I have, at many moments, wanted to give up. I feel more desperate than ever to give students who want to become analysts some assurance that there is a good, reasonable path to achieve their professional aims, and this desperation has only contributed to my break in will. What future?

I give this grim diagnosis precisely because I have more conviction in what psychoanalysis can do, maybe even more than most others, never once wanting to dilute the name: *psychoanalyst*. I say this loving what is peculiar about the profession, to say nothing of the respect I have for what I have come to know intimately about human suffering and our shared impasses. Psychoanalysis cannot lapse into an anxious collective fantasy about itself but must meet the world holding onto what is unique in its cure: a courage for conversion without promise or pity. One more time: Who has the courage?

CONVERSION

So, it is within this peculiar situation of psychoanalysis that I happened upon the word *conversion*, not only as a question concerning the kind of quasi-religious turning point in the strange life of a psychoanalyst—the move from analysand to psychoanalyst, from psychoanalyst to training analyst—but also as what psychoanalysis is founded on. Freud stumbled upon conversion when listening to supposedly sick women in early-twentieth-century Vienna, showing that it was possible for nothing more than speaking to alter the body and psyche. Conversion, then, is not only the cause of psychoanalysis but also its desired effect, so that the founding of a discipline and the action of that discipline were inextricably linked through this term. All these aspects of conversion are equivalent in some rigorous way.

Might an investigation into this knot bring psychoanalysis into the present, stretched between the passing of a religious age, through modernity, into the delirium of twenty-first-century life? What can conversion, from the perspective of a psychoanalyst, tell us about today? Religious conversion is certainly bound up with a psychoanalytic sense of conversion and should not be dismissed as entirely different nor seen as part of a distant illusory past. Work must be done on the interactions between these terms, historically and theoretically; Freud's dismissal of religion is too facile. Since we live in a time considered to be a return to religious dogmatism, accompanied by a craving for spiritual transformation, religious conversion cannot simply be tossed aside. The therapeutic era is more bound up with this religious return than we like to think.[3]

Conversion disorder is also linked to psychosomatic concerns, which are generally accused of being "false" illnesses and pain, hypochondria the obvious culprit. I want to suspend this hasty equivalence. The tie to the question of the body is central to my work, central to the term, but we must first ask questions about this body before assuming anything about the nature of a psychosomatic illness. Psychosomatic questions concern the totality of the organism, meaning that it is affected in total—this interplay being inherent to religious conversion, this inside-out action that William James emphasized in his work and that, in many personal accounts by mystics, is a transformation always more of the body than simply spiritual.[4]

The term "conversion" suggests overturning, a process of subversion; the Latin *convertere* means to turn and re-turn. To be affected on the material and physical plane is also to ask a question about affect or about the affects involved in conversion. Thinking about what it means to be affected, to be moved by a constant stream of affects, introduces a play between subject and object through the question of the body. One is struck as an object, from the outside, as a body, even when the conversion in question is seen as the apex of subjective change—who one will come to be as opposed to what one was before. There is a funny paradox here between conversion linked to inner experience and something that—at least phenomenologically, if not structurally—is best described as taking place on or from the outside. This is to say nothing of questions of will, for what part of a conversion can even begin to be described as linked to a set of decisive conscious actions? Through the question of affect, the body insists.

We cannot escape what concerns both the individual, the special species of subjectivity that is sought in using this term conversion, and the inhuman, mechanical, objectifying language of the sheer momentum and movement implied by the process. This renders conversion both an isolated moment in time, a turning point, and a live wire that is touched again and again in order to produce the supposed change. At any historical moment in the term's deployment we can glimpse new modes of linking terms that have remained divided—inner and outer, subject and object, soma and psyche, point and line.

This book is not some hymn to the unity of the human, body and soul, or to a unity of the human and the environment, enthralled by some idea of a naturalistic order. Rather, conversion, mapped in this way, pinpoints a pressure felt around division and unity or order and disorder. This brings me to the title of this work: *Conversion Disorder*. In what follows, I will give a more detailed history of the term from Freud to the present. For now, it suffices to say that "conversion disorder" is a diagnosis that is part of the subgroup "somatic symptoms and related disorders," which includes hypochondria, pain disorder, and somatic symptom disorder (APA 2013). Conversion requires a neurological evaluation of symptoms that can range from dizziness to loss of consciousness to changes in motor or sensory functions, from difficulty seeing, smelling, and touching to paralysis, weakness or numbness in the body, and even difficulty speaking or swallowing. The diagnosis gives a nod to psychoanalytic history, the link between the first conception of psychoanalysis and the vicissitudes of neurology, something that was a source of contention in the last edition of the *Diagnostic and Statistical Manual of Mental Disorders*. Many felt it should go the way of hysteria, which disappeared in the 1980s.

Freud uses conversion hysteria and hysteria interchangeably, though "hysteria" in its later iterations came to denote a set of structural issues other than symptomatic conversion. What conversion disorder retains of hysteria, unlike the other somatoform disorders, is the lack of anxiety that accompanies its bodily symptoms. They are not a source of constant preoccupation, as they are in hypochondria, pain disorder, and somatic symptom disorder, all of which produce abnormal thoughts, feelings, and behaviors in response to distressing somatic symptoms. In conversion disorder, the symptom is there—glaring even—but it is oddly unattended to by the patient. This is why it is linked to dissociation, alexithymia, or depersonalization: a splitting of the subject. For Freud, the *belle indifférence* of the hysteric shows the force of repression and the power of the symptom, in particular to free the mind from anxiety or mental preoccupations.

I like the two words together, "conversion" and "disorder," implying that conversion in itself is neither a simple disorder nor a simple hysteria. A sense lingers that there is a hidden order in conversion beyond or behind all its disarray. Conversion keeps its potential power in reserve, a power alive and unpacifiable, a power that twists and turns and wreaks havoc. Perhaps this is why it is capable of remaining on the books despite this young field's many fluctuations. Perhaps this is why conversion is about being able to slip into the provinces of the body, almost without notice. The other somatoform disorders—and hysteria, too—are too noisy, circumscribed, and suspect. Conversion, on the other hand, rearranges the pieces on the board, changes their function, and refuses to expend its energy on the distractions of anxiety.

This does not mean that the everyday symptomatic concerns of the body should not be linked to the question of conversion. I'm certainly aware of these, and their proliferating insistences are at the core of why I turned to this topic. The body has always been one of the most important markers in analysis. It makes its presence felt at every moment, especially since it can also do so by virtue of its absence. Speech deprived of body, the patient on the couch like a corpse, always alerts the analyst to a problem, even simply by virtue of the boredom or sleepiness this lifelessness exerts upon their listening ear. The vacillations in the affective life of the body carry an analysis along or grind it to a halt.

If I survey my practice, everyone is troubled by what it means to have a body, having a series of bodily symptoms that define their life. Much of the everyday increasingly takes place via assimilation: life tailored to the demands of work, self-promotion, and lifestyle, ironized, mediated, and distanced, on the one hand, and, on the other, shot through with sentimental and aggressive claims to authentic experience. The body rebels first. Even when lifestyle tries to cater to this body in protest—like the streamlining of diet, exercise (usually something like yoga or Pilates), and meditation, along with a generalized ethos of well-being—something doesn't sit right. We do not know what to do with this body of ours at a time when the demands made upon it exceed the vicissitudes of physical exertion. It breaks, along with the ability to feel or be reassured by pleasure.

Patients have difficulty speaking to this predicament, tending to use the diffuse but strident voice of anxiety for quite a long time before finding a means of addressing the specificity of their situation. They take pressures and pains and protests in the body personally, meaning that they assume a kind of guilt in relation to their existence. It's their fault, just like the failure to achieve wealth, success, fame, beauty, and even orgasm is their fault. From within this stagnant economy of culpability (one that easily reverses into blame at other moments) you can find the deep longing for a way out, for another way of life, including a way to find the conviction to pursue something other than what has been offered—this I also want to name conversion.

Conversion disorder as linked to the body is often associated with a kind of immediacy, concreteness, or dogmatism—I'm sick because I'm sick—which is pitted against the delay implied by the act of thinking and reflecting. While this is certainly one of our contemporary ills—dogmatism requires very little thought—nevertheless, conversion disorder teaches us that thought is not necessarily the antidote to the doctrinaire. One of the wagers of this work is that by addressing the question of the body in the conversion process of psychoanalysis, knowing the weight and pressure of maintaining any link to the life of the body, we can ease a path through the deadlock between the suspension implied in thinking and the carelessness of immediacy. The bodily symptom has the potential to structure this divide differently.

Another wager, so characteristically psychoanalytic, is that wrestling with the body means dealing with the sexual. Any deadlock in psychoanalysis is first and foremost sexual in nature—the very language of tension concerns this drive-ridden erogenous body. We must ask what Freud or psychoanalysis more generally means by the sexual—a question I intend to exhaust, if possible. In focusing specifically on the body and sexuality, I avoid the vicissitudes of gender and its social construction more than I have in the past, and perhaps more than I am comfortable with doing. Here, I assert something primary about what it means to live with a body and with sexual drives and what these have to do with conversion or radical change.

I have come to the conclusion that what is important is not what a body demonstrates or speaks, that is, making the body a question of translation or interpretation. Many see analysis as a constant process of translating this body into language. The question of conversion has taught me that we need to move differently. I have come to see in this body a surface that holds a degree of sexual tension that begins to define what it even means to speak; that is, the body and its particular relationship to the unconscious change the nature of discourse, not vice versa. Psychoanalytic work is embedded in discourse that nonetheless manages to touch this sexual body and change what it is possible to do, no less feel. This is why I invoke the insane tautology in psychoanalysis that conversion must be subject to conversion.[5]

There is one truth I have found as an analyst: I must follow this body. I must follow the drive as it appears in a session, pushing toward some place or point unknown to either me or the patient, which produces the utmost tension in a treatment. This act of following creates more friction than any deconstructive work, any genealogical deduction, any intersubjective moment of contact or empathy. I do not discount these. But my faith is in the circuit of a treatment as bound to this stamp of the body that appears in critical moments, fuels the transference, and moves in the direction of its own dissolution. The so-called desire for psychoanalysis must be assumed by the one who directs the analysis in this way, with the impropriety of this attention to the body. Even to begin to be able to set the stage for this kind of work with a specific client is a cardinal achievement. I follow you in order to extinguish myself there.

Even Freud threw up his hands in the face of conversion—something he named too obscure to continue working with—turning back to anxiety (as failed conversion) and effectively throwing the concept into erasure. Conversion will only happen at the limit, and you walk into this terrain without knowing what, or when, or how, or even why. I ask this of my readers as much as I ask it of my patients because it is here that the weight of conversion rests. The transference will carry you forward, or it won't. And if it doesn't, you probably should go elsewhere. You don't ask why something has grabbed you—what takes you in is simply a fact—this or that conversion. To ask is already an undoing of the force of the act, much as Freud said that to be neurotic was simply to ask why, to ask about the meaning of existence.

This backsliding is a moment I live through on a daily basis with patients. Sometimes it just isn't possible to proceed any further with me; I understand the pressure and the about-face. Something can be said, vigorously, that had not been said before. It is registered by me. I imagine, perhaps wrongly, that it is heard by the patient as well. It feels like a moment of breath in a terse exchange. In this space, I am sometimes met with their unrelenting *why*, their request for an explanation that can extend into the future—why and so what and now what, as if I could simply answer these questions. The moment, the act of saying something now, is foreclosed, which I mean in the strong sense of the term: It is abolished.

I find this closure unbearable, which I feel in my body. It builds up on the periphery like storm walls or a beachhead threatened by the sea. I try to shed some of this at the end of the day, to chip away at so much lost opportunity, at so much given away. As an analyst I feel exhausted by everything that is allowed to return to helpless and impotent requests or the harsh outlines of guilt and self-laceration: letting one's words slip or, better yet, handing oneself over to an aggression that wants to knock over the pieces on the gameboard—directed at me in countless demands, fits, and hateful investigations of my person. I take none of this personally; I like being attacked—it feels more alive than depressive lethargy and obsessive emptying out. But it does bruise the analytic body.

One becomes an analyst because one believes in the power of openings, of reversals and revelations, of breaks in a system that can create new sensualities, new symptomatic configurations. But one also becomes an analyst because one believes in repetition, in trauma, in defense, in entrenchment. Caught between these two, where else will all this be felt than in the body of the analyst, which is met as an open or closed conduit? In what other profession must one remain at this threshold—and for so long? And finally, what in the conversion of the analyst makes bearing this at all possible? What if the answer is—nothing? Nothing in your personal analysis prepares you for this kind of work. Nothing tells you how much you will have to take on, how difficult it is to live through so many other lives, to have them live in your body. They do live there. All the conversions in a treatment happen because of this living.

THE SUIT

The patient walks in, and you suddenly, seemingly for no reason, wonder if she's pregnant. Maybe it's the way she's dressed today? Then you pause; you realize this would really be out of the blue and even stranger if you'd guessed correctly. Maybe it's a wish. The soundness of imputing a wish seems worse than imputing a reality. Is it? Bits and pieces of the last session flash through your mind, nothing that really paves the way for this strange thought. You wonder whether you have lost your mind—this really is the intrusion of *your* wish—and then, unresolved, you return to listening. Strangely enough, you tune in at the moment that you realize she has had the most important dream of her analysis this year, and it is centered on the figure of pregnancy—not pregnancy as such, but pregnancy as what two people can put into one another's bodies.

The word "suit" looms large, not only as the clothes one wears or, in her case, what she doesn't wear (rushing in are all her questions about her career) but also suit as what fits, what suits a person, when another knows how to buy you clothes (so rare!), and this nagging unresolved question of what she should be or do, also what she should feel. On the other side of this emerges an ominous figure, suit as a legal case, with all the vicissitudes of blame and guilt, what is passed down from one generation to another. This is the question in her analysis and the hinge of her deep depression.

To have had this dream, you realize as you listen to her, is already to be moving away from this legalistic order that dispenses judgment (I never wanted to judge her—it was incredibly hard to be in this place she put me for so long). Locating herself somewhere new, somewhere depression won't be so threatening, is about to happen because she hears the difference between suit, suit, and suit. This word speaks to her transference, where she is in it and where it is about to shift. The suit is also a question about the difference between parents and analysts, parents who put things into your body and analysts who let you reside in theirs in order to take some things back and perhaps to leave others.

All the turn-of-the-century interest in telepathy by psychoanalysts—the fascinating question of unconscious communication; the contemporary talk of what is called the "intersubjective third," which means something about the space where ideas and affects take shape between analyst and patient; and even everything that can be classed under the heading of countertransference—is about what it means to have these two bodies in such intimate proximity in an act of listening. We listen in a way that takes on the body, the drives, the unconscious, and the vicissitudes of sexuality rather than quiet them, which is what everyday chit-chat does—glosses it, tames it, and, if it can, brings this body down to a whisper. I do not discount the huge backlog of literature on this topic, but I want to approach the question not on the basis of pathology, technique, or even metapsychology but through the lived life of the analyst, perhaps my life lived as an analyst, with this body, these patients, in this impossible profession as it exists now.

What did I know when I allowed this strange thought to emerge regarding pregnancy, a thought that foreshadowed my patient's dream? There is nothing mystical here—probably she was dressed a little more maternally and held her body differently because she had the dream, which I picked up on. I've been working with her for six years. I know her yet have no experience of her outside this room. I register something the minute I look at her face, or see how she puts her bag down, or whether she's chosen to go to the bathroom before a session. This is the level on which we live with our patients, something much more difficult to do in everyday life without the frame of the office, the frame of free association, or the frame simply of psychoanalysis.

That the frame can allow this attention is its importance, not as a protection akin to the rule of abstinence or professional boundaries. The frame allows you to live with, and so read, your patients. It is folly to think that this reading is easily done; it requires discipline and repetition, the momentum of work so that a sequence—both temporal and spatial—can develop in order for the analyst to direct a treatment. Freud called this the architecture of an analysis, and it mirrors the hysterical architecture of the symptom. Putting the two together, forcing them to resonate, is how psychoanalysis works.

KNOWLEDGE

What kind of knowledge, then, is the knowledge of the psychoanalyst? And what role does knowledge play in conversion disorder? It is an understatement to say that I have a fundamental distrust of knowledge in its many guises. There is too much of it around, and it doesn't seem to do a whole lot. The importance of knowledge cannot be disregarded, but I have witnessed its problematic effects consistently overshadowing its positive ones. Like anyone else, I am susceptible to wanting to be in the know. One might imagine that it would be better to speak of wisdom, which would be fine with me if the term wasn't so reified and easily misunderstood, susceptible to the arrogance of a sage master. I also don't feel all that wise.

As a psychoanalyst, I've consistently been witness to how little knowledge makes a life better, how symptomatic it can be, and—in the worst of situations—how it winds its way toward a sustainable delirium. This is to say nothing of how aggressively it is often deployed, knowledge devolving into sheer argument for the sake of argument: the problem with elitism. I say that I feel forced because this wasn't where I wanted to end up. I am a child of the Enlightenment as much as any of us are. But what I experience as an analyst is that knowing clouds listening. The territory of knowledge, expectation, does not solve the problems that analysis is trying to work with. In fact, it usually makes them worse.

Lacan said that psychoanalysis takes place by listening between the clouds, nodding to Aristophanes's play. *The Clouds* is about a fight to the death between an old corrupt philosophical Platonism and new-age sophistry, a battle between the older and the younger generation. One lays claim to the truth, a truth one wants to conserve without being required to abide by it or produce from it a prescriptive ethical system. The other has given up completely on this conundrum in hatred of the hypocrisy of this older generation, deciding that whatever takes the form of a winning argument will be considered the truth and will decide the course of action.

The play satirically winds its way toward the tragic consequences of a complete breakdown between these warring partners—the sophist setting fire to Socrates's school with him and all his students inside, leaving them to die in a blazing ruin. The only opening in this strange play (which is supposed to be a comedy) seems to be in the impersonal chorus of clouds and their mechanistic cycles of amassing, exploding, and clearing off. They are like the living thought of libidinal cycles, ones that are shown to be—at the very least—beyond the hubris of personal belief and civil war, and they have an air of feminine sensuality to them. Truth gives the appearance of being the source, what emerges from the clouds, but this is just an effect; the two—truth and clouds—are always found together. The clouds hold the point of conversion like rain, showing that it is not a property of either philosophy or knowledge but of a process.

"Listen. The Clouds are a saturate water solution. Tumescence in motion, of necessity, produces precipitation. When these distended masses collide— boom! Fulmination" (Aristophanes *Clouds* 383), says Socrates. Strepsiades immediately asks, "But who makes them move before they collide? Isn't that Zeus?" Socrates answers, "Not Zeus, idiot. The convection-principle!" Aristophanes has Socrates say there is no Zeus, no god, but only these three pathways—great chaos, the clouds, and bamboozle! Of the three, the clouds have movement, a life, and a logic, including the force of destiny that forces men to bow before them in humility. Not a god, he says, but perhaps like a goddess.

Important for Lacan in this parable is that we not give in to the desire to force a clearing. This will only end in bamboozle or chaos. We have to listen between clouds—something material is suspended there. *The Clouds* appears in Lacan's 1970–1971 seminar *On a Discourse That Might Not Be a Semblance* at the moment that he seeks to contrast discourse with writing, searching for something more real than just the blah blah blah of discourse. Writing, for Lacan, is not the same as knowledge or speaking; writing, when it produces significant effects, does not contribute to knowledge but rather ruptures it, placing conversion disorder on this terrain of convection. This very real act of disordering knowledge, overturning it, challenges our self-conception, our idea of truth. The question of the body is increasingly foregrounded by the question of writing—it is the material that is suspended there, that amasses, explodes, rains down, dissipates once again, and in this process writes itself into the earth.

This sexual body will always be kept in suspension, away from knowledge, even when it is its object. This, Lacan says, is what Freud taught us. In Freud's *Three Essays on the Theory of Sexuality* ([1905c] 1995), he speaks about the sexual research of children and concludes that their efforts are "habitually fruitless" and end in a renunciation that leaves behind "a permanent injury to the instinct for knowledge" (7:197). All this is carried out in complete solitude and leaves you, once again, in solitude. Nevertheless, it is—according to Freud—an important disenchantment, "a first step towards taking an independent attitude in the world," and it implies a "high degree of alienation" of the child from the people in his world "who formerly enjoyed his complete confidence" (7:197). Knowledge runs up against the limit of a sexuality it can neither contain nor order. Sexuality is first a source of alienation and then a source, hopefully, of separation. What the clouds represent in Aristophanes, situated away from the dimension of human hubris, knowledge, and generational drama, points to the possibility of separation by virtue of touching this essence of the sexual.

SEPARATION

This brings me to an unexpected trope that emerged when writing this book about conversion: namely, separation. We might say that it is in refusing to separate truth and clouds, body and language—refusing to seek for one behind or before the other—that another vision of separation began to emerge. This vision is not separation as individualization, nor is it a concept of truth or self-knowledge. Separation is a quality that is attached to what it means to have a body that leads to an encounter with what it is impossible to know—in particular about sexuality, bodies, identity. Evoking this body in analysis, in all of its sexual pleasures and pains, brings the fact of separation to bear. This is what writes itself in and through the psychoanalytic process, dragging us toward the final moment: termination.

Psychoanalysis has always circled this theme. It can be found in the vogue for what is called "attachment theory," following the development of a child's experience of separation anxiety. Attachment, or a secure base, is code for being able to tolerate separateness, though it has given birth to all kinds of manuals for "attachment-style" parenting that tell you, paradoxically, never to leave your child. The idea of separation is also at the heart of most ideas concerning autonomy in the wake of ego psychology, including its opposing camp, the relational theories, with their emphasis on mutuality as an attempt to correct what was too individualistic about mainstream American psychoanalysis. Whether one has autonomy or can engage from this autonomy in mutuality, the emphasis is on the achievement of a kind of separateness. As well, the Kleinian notion of the depressive position speaks to the solitude of separateness and the mournful regret for what was done to the other before this psychic achievement.

The difficulty I have with so much of this literature is that it speaks about separation, tells us about what this separation is, and makes us vulnerable not only to the problems of knowledge but to the moralism that is its twin. Many of the ethical atrocities committed in the history of psychoanalysis happened because of this edict to separate: Be who you are! Separate! It is as if we failed to find ourselves separate enough to know not to decry or command anyone. Separation is a process; it is always something half-done in us and cannot be judged by an observer like one might measure distance.

Measurement is always ideal; when you delineate the supposedly ideal position of the other, you are immediately caught playing an endless game of too close, too far—a collapse of separation if there ever was one. To say that the operation is formal means that it is not about placing yourself in the right position or deciding on the right distance but rather creating something that overhauls the entire system of measurement. This process is itself a conversion, in the same way that a conversion is a change in scale, size, or dimension or a change in substance, as in chemistry. There is *this* possibility of change, yet the clouds still do not go away. Psychoanalysis, conversion, and separation—like the clouds—are an unending process. This is what is lived out in the transference, no different from any other love, something that forces us to begin to read between the lines, to let the rain fall upon burning soil.

I am reminded of a dream where a loved other was packing his bags to leave and zipped the zipper, something that at that very moment I felt in my body on its midline. The dream was surrounded by the vicissitudes of jealousy—he was leaving for another—and the two affects were tied together at this hinge of felt separation. Jealousy is simply an acknowledgment of the fact of separation, like the pain of one's body closed upon itself. There is room here for desire, always desire for the other's body, but it leaves us at their mercy, wounded like Freud's child.

I don't know how autonomy or even mutuality measures up in this dream, except maybe as a point of hope or even a fantasy. The cloudy outlines of depression and anxiety are more clear somehow, along with the necessity for constantly confronting them, trying to move across the pull they exert on the surface of a body. Zip also implies the need to move quickly, especially if the other is on his or her way out. There isn't time to hesitate. There isn't anything more to understand. Do you want the other to leave or not? What is the attachment?

What is fascinating to me about psychic life, especially the dreams one has so late in the game, is that this bedrock refusal of separation simply won't go away. If Freud was optimistic about the solitude of a child's research, it is an optimism that isn't mirrored in the world around us—meaning I do not see the invention of new or better ways of living separation but rather its continued collapse or disavowal. My patients, especially the most alone, the most isolated, struggle with separation because the choice of solitude is made in order to escape the conundrum, not confront it. Indeed, most bodily symptoms bear the trace of a failed separation going back to childhood, like the stomachaches that could keep you home from school. If Freud was suspicious of love (which he thinks of as a species of madness and illusion), there is more hope I would place on its side for throwing us into the fire, for showing us how little—despite work or success or life lived—we escape of ourselves and our history, and for how difficult being together is on the basis of this fact of separation.

IMPOSSIBLE

So the task of this book is to ask about psychoanalysis, this impossible profession, with these themes that converge around the word *conversion*. Can this work have a place? Is there room for conversion as conceived by psychoanalysis? Can we think of psychoanalysis as conversion in the most general sense that Freud gave to this term, namely, "the psychophysical aptitude for transposing large quantities of energy"? I think we must ask these questions of psychoanalysis anew, ask them in a world that loves the massive scale of quantification as the language of justification; a world where symptoms have gone viral, like antibiotic-resistant bacteria; a world where the contradiction of hankering for instantaneous fame takes place in a generation that stays at home longer than ever, hooked into a virtual life. We must ask about psychoanalysis in the face of a generation that lives in the contradiction of mental illness as both a pestilence and a status, a national crisis and a cherished identity, one that might *even* bring fame, like being on *Hoarders* or in rehab.

With this army of impasses, we can look closely at what the world today tells us about why psychoanalysis seems so arduous, if not dangerous, in its anachronism. The book moves in this fashion, tracing a circuit from philosophical discourse to psychoanalytic theory, to the exploration of cases and personal diaristic musings, elucidating something of the continued life of a psychoanalyst. It does this in order to map a certain experience of this terrain, one I think of as psychoanalytic in its essence, insofar as it is a terrain that moves, shifts, slips, turns around, and escapes. The book decamps in a space between the personal and the impersonal, the historical and the fanciful or fictive, and the pathos of confession and the attempt at rigorous investigation. Conversion thrives in this tension of topography, in this ambiguity of passage.

These questions might seem directed to a closed audience, for the analysts better to situate themselves—and who cares, if it is an insider's dilemma?—but I don't believe that this is a question asked only for us. The place of analytic discourse in the wider world is unique. Our strange moment of invention remains crucial to our continuing story, unable to shake off the tie to Freud or the peculiar aspects of our institutional life. This is the story of psychoanalysis as a plague, the eternal resistance to it and all that hyperbole, but it is also its strange amalgamation of historical forms: one part medicine, one part religion, one part cult, another part philosophy, another part art, another part science. Psychoanalysis is the repeated attempt to stage its own life while never being in the right place at the right time.

Does this widen the potential audience for this little thought experiment? This book is an attempt to meet those who have questions about the field and what makes psychoanalysis specifically what it is. It does so with an assemblage of discourses, transposing the question of conversion across the field of psychoanalysis from the most general theoretical explications in Freud and Lacan to the most intimate details of a clinical case, across disciplines from history to social theory to philosophy, and across the individual question of what it means to be a psychoanalyst toward the future of the psychoanalytic institution. Always holding the idea of conversion in mind in its many valences, it is also the labor of an author attempting to speak to a personal version of conversion, the attempt to overcome my doubts about the profession or, more specifically, my ability to handle the work. In this way, it asks the reader not only to identify with the author for the short time span of reading but also to put this identification to work in a terrain loosely called *psychoanalysis*. In some sense, it asks you to find within yourself your own disordered conversion.

At this frontier, the figure of conversion is formally enacted, forcing the reader to move across so many territories, transposing a constellation of thoughts from one place to another, shifting their identification from personal experience and narrative to that of the another, and then to so many others, to find out how to live with all this. This assemblage moves through a landscape of thoughts, dreams, stories, and theories, forcing the question of transposition, which Freud says we must find the aptitude for. Perhaps we can translate aptitude here as courage. So, to my readers, if you've made it this far, if you've picked up this book, thumbed its pages, read the back cover or even this introduction, then take me at my word when I say: Being a psychoanalyst is impossible, more impossible than ever, yet I am a psychoanalyst. I want to tell you about the breaking point I'm at and what that has to do with being a psychoanalyst in the twenty-first century.

The first chapter of this book will trace the definition of conversion culturally, philosophically, and psychoanalytically, circling the territory that defines the project. Moving between Freud and Lacan around the question of the body and language, the body and sexuality, I increasingly speak to my difficulties as a practicing analyst. I then move to a reading of the term "conversion" in Freud going back to his self-analysis, work on etiology and diagnosis, and the first therapeutic encounter with hysterical patients. Importantly, Freud's willing erasure of the term "conversion" in his 1926 work *Inhibitions, Symptoms, and Anxiety* shows a fundamental encounter with the enigma of bodily transformation. This leads into writing more personal in tone, asking what dreams can tell us about conversion, alongside an interrogation of psychoanalytic others working on this precipice. This chapter moves between a series of dreams mixed with fables from the psychoanalytic ether.

Next, Freud's essay "The Taboo on Virginity" holds center stage as a means of speaking to a question about sexual inhibition and sexual anesthesia as a specific kind of conversion disorder, linking this to a number of cultural analyses by Freud that mirror many of the first chapters' contemporary concerns. The virginity essay speaks to why women and feminine sexuality are so central to any question of conversion not only clinically but in terms of our broader questions about the organization of civilization. Here the question of conversion hinges on the birth of sexuality and the problems of love and marriage. The book then moves on to reflections concerning the label of "hysteria," especially its supposed disappearance as a psychiatric entity. I turn to manifestations of hysteria in literature and end with several cases in order to claim that conversion is a better name, especially in its capacity to speak to the "hysterical" desire for change and the establishment of new social ties and ways of speaking.

The book then takes a philosophical turn, reading Giorgio Agamben's work as speaking to a question concerning conversion. Agamben's historical and philosophical archeology aims at exposing a more original libidinal economy—what Freud and Lacan would call the drive. Through Agamben I hope to convey a different picture of the history of conversion, including the part that religious and economic conversions play in the history of the psychoanalytic institution. I then move into a detailed analysis of Freud and Lacan on the question of anxiety and separation, playing with the theme of "coitus interruptus" not as the stopping of orgasm that Freud mistakenly believed caused anxiety neurosis but as the attempt to bring the drive to a halt at the place where separation is experienced. What these two readings—one philosophical, one psychoanalytic—illuminate is a theme that has been present all along: namely, how conversion is seeking not merely a transformation but an act of radical separation or division.

Still lingering in the province of philosophy, a quick chapter on three thinkers—Bachelard, Nancy, and Foucault—who articulate this theme of disorder and separation through the figures of fire, touch, and madness. These three meditations lead to reconsideration of how to think what is inside and outside, the relation between body and language, and the importance of sense or nonsense. The processes of radical exteriorization, blocking of sense, and separation are illustrated in two longer case studies: one of child and one of a woman. I see these cases as a kind of dividing line in the book, for what follows turns to the role of the psychoanalyst, their position in the work, and the conversion of the patient into an analyst proper.

From this vantage point, we have a chapter on the drive and the impossible position of the analyst—a position that can only be found through a conversion experience in one's analysis. In the experience of tracing one's drive, the body emerges as the ground zero of analytic work and analytic cure. What follows is a reading of Freud's late paper "On the Subtleties of a Faulty Action" and Lacan's late seminar *Encore*, looking at how conversion has led to a variety of failures in psychoanalysis institutionally. Both Freud and Lacan can be seen as searching in their end days for a conversion in relation to their audiences. Finally, there is a reading of Lacan's paper "Variations on the Standard Treatment," where he asks: What changes in a psychoanalysis that allows the patient to become an analyst, and what role does the analyst's analysis continue to play? This last chapter concludes with a short case that illuminates the place of a symptom in my self-analysis, showing how this symptom plays a role in the analyst's listening.

I

DAYBREAK

Ashamed of having gone dizzy and unconscious in order to do something that I would never again know how I had done—since doing it I had removed myself from all participation. I had not wanted "to know."

—CLARICE LISPECTOR, *THE PASSION ACCORDING TO G.H.*

DAYBREAK

I had not wanted to know. I still don't want to know. We inhabit a body that is not an object of knowledge unless it wants to become the object of science, in which case it ceases to be ours. One is, as it were, under investigation or inquiry. Try the other side of the coin. The mind, in the case of epistemological questions—What do we know? How do we know what we know?—enters into a reflexive loop that never quite catches up to itself, a search that can grow quickly lifeless too. My typing fingers know more, or know without knowing what they are doing, because more than anything, they are involved in an act of writing. My desire is allowed to enter back into the game, if even only a little. What did I want in wanting, or not wanting, to know anything in the first place?

Nothing kills desire faster than pinning it to what I can only call "knowledge," draining from it a force that gives it body, however momentary or enigmatic. I don't want to fetishize immediacy; rather, it is a question of finding a way forward. Knowledge, taken as a system of meaning, meets with the unity of self-justification. It never arrives without a little bit of justification, the need to feel one's feet firmly on the ground. This march of progress brings with it an impious air of authority. At least, we might say, there are feet; those little feet that don't make a sound or the hard thump of laboring feet—those aren't mine. So, the body makes its appearance in parts, as part of the desire to know or not know.

I have a dream that I can one day find the way to get rid of everything that I think I know, that I might be able to begin again. It is a regressive dream, or a dream of regression—the search for fresh eyes—like the inverse face of a world that likes to think of evolution as some kind of learning curve on a path toward mastery. Progress sounds to me like waiting to plateau, to find even ground and finally stand still, imagining that was progress. Reactively, I'm trying to walk backward on my hands—equally as silly, I agree, but perhaps there is a less pessimistic or less reactive idea of regression than simply the idea of backsliding away from rationality. For Freud, the question of knowledge was always a question of sexual curiosity, and sexuality, he suggests, never moves in straight lines, never moves this curiosity straightforwardly. Libido folds in on itself, or it simply exists as a series of folds, sometimes found in the form of a striving to know, to make something of itself, the object of discovery, one among many variations of autoeroticism, this folding as a folding back or in upon the self.

We try to master ourselves, self-regulate our access to pleasure, defend against pleasure that has grown too intense—a losing game if there ever was one—but it is a first and necessary attempt at having our body be our body. The body doesn't easily submit to this effort, nor does it bend well to the displacement away from the erotic in the direction of knowledge. From the fluttering joy of inquiry, to the coursing anxiety of the search for meaning, to the pained investigation of what might be expected of us, this research grows more and more serious. As Lacan once said, "we don't know whether the series is the source of the serious" (1972, 26). On the surface, he is asking a question about his endless series of seminars, asking what on earth he is doing there, teaching again. But it is also a question about the series of sexual objects that shape human life, a whole bodily history. "Secrete sense vigorously and you'll see how much more easy life becomes!" Lacan yells to his audience, whom he disdains for wanting common sense, which he says does not exist (1972, 35). Sexuality, the body, he claims, deprives us of this. Yet if one secretes sense—making it a vigorous product of the body—life, he says, will become easier!

The child immediately feels that its body is not up to the task of what it has stumbled upon when it stumbles upon itself. Jubilation first, fragility second. The mechanisms of identification follow, set upon the one who seems to know or at least seems up to it in the eyes of this child. The loved other is now in a position to provide answers, answers that carry in them the rules that map the child's surround. The child wasn't originally looking for rules—but there they are, the adults, asking you to bend yourself to their will. In this unfolding series of misunderstandings, this confusion of tongues,[1] it is hard to imagine how to keep anything alive, to retain that first trace of excitement in the face of so much that demands vigilance—keeping us on our toes, gridding our existence. The desire for mastery is finally overturned, leaving the child at the mercy of something ever further on the outside.

For many, anxiety means beating a retreat to the shelter of imagination, which is still, when all is said and done, a permutation of knowledge. Perhaps imagination is the shape that knowledge takes when left too much on the inside. Nevertheless, knowledge and imagination do not occupy the same space. They are differently folded, outside in or inside out. Imagination, in a sense, doesn't look to occupy anything other than the field of attention, usually coming underfoot, at play, unoccupied. I cannot inhabit my imagination. Try as I may, I don't have my imagination. Then who does? That is as good a place to begin as any, and it happens to be the place that psychoanalysis begins, my occupation of sorts.

What this occupation tells me is that what is on the inside we can keep, though we cannot ultimately have it, and what is on the outside we can have, though it will never be anything that will feel ours. A strange dilemma. "What is at stake here [in the psychoanalytic act] is something like a conversion in the position which results for the subject regarding what is involved in his relation to knowledge. How can we not immediately admit that there cannot but be established a really dangerous gap if only some people take an adequate view of this subversion" (Lacan 1967–1968, 16).[2] Does this conversion always appear marked by negation, in particular the negation of knowledge, the "I do not know," while nevertheless demanding that we find a way to get to know it—in the biblical sense?

Foucault described dreams thus: "the world on the daybreak of its first explosion, when it still coincided with its own existence" (1993, 45). This perhaps should be contrasted with his vision of the future found in his short, beautiful essay "Madness, the Absence of Work" (1995), where insanity says nothing by inhabiting a space of pure rationality. Language, he imagines, will have folded around itself so completely that it will be uninterrupted even by madness. Immanence, Foucault writes, would be absolutely visible but empty, not even anything worth striving for. This infinite search ends in a rather alarming nowhere: "In the eyes of some unknown culture—one quite possibly already quite near—we shall be those that have come closest to those sentences never really pronounced, those two sentences equally contradictory and impossible as the famous 'I am lying' and both pointing to the same empty self-reference: 'I am writing' and 'I am delirious'" (1995, 297).

We move from the explosive coincidence of dream to a final divergence in the absence of work or insanity. We no longer move, he says, from the full to the empty or from the empty to the full but live between two impossible and impossibly filled-in figures. Madness for Foucault is the human without the possibility of dreaming—this work of daybreak—equivalent to the absence of madness in the uselessness of pure self-reference, what he calls a seamless surface of knowledge that renders language unworkable.

Giving up on knowledge felt like a revelation, a first explosion; something fell out between thought and speech or between me and the investigation of me. This is only a momentary phenomenon; thus it is also an ongoing battle. But as far as I can see, it is the battle of the psychoanalyst in the face of a demand that they be the ones who finally know, this haste on the side of the patient, and the exigency of the demand to make known what cannot be held in the container called knowledge. And isn't this always the fantasy about the analyst? The force that sews people's mouths shut when you announce what you do? And if the analyst was to stand in this place, find themselves there, would this not be the real madness: the absence of work? Yes, yet . . . this demand is also the earnest and gentle inquiry of any patient who makes their way into an analyst's office—What can I find out here? What I can I know?

Coaches or pundits or teachers or talking heads readily assume their place in the Agora, the field of *doxa*, as unending opinions or articles of faith held in the pews of a church or bound by the edge of what we consider a sanctuary, even when virtual. The virtual, burdened by so much information—it's hard to know how it all holds together for anyone—almost feels at a breaking point. Almost. It has always been the case that the "almost," the precariousness of any edge, inspires a certain kind of pull upon the reins. The almost makes you feel the bit inside your mouth, and you dig your heels in. The psychoanalyst joins the chorus of voices, and, indeed, a thousand therapies beckon—competing cures in a bustling marketplace. There is no one to recommend any one thing. Care is reduced to the pitch of a salesman and feels ever more anonymous. "I am a psychoanalyst!" they scream.

I prefer to think of my vocation as a psychoanalyst as a quiet liturgy to the power of the symptom, to this intimate world where very little information can be given, even when there is so much to say. Inside this multitude, I see one of the greatest of intimacies on offer—one I know daily in the demand turned upon me by a patient who needs me to know something. *Needs me to. With urgency.* With great shame, I return this demand to them, even if I supply a placeholder, a stopgap, given to ease the anxiety that hurtles through their flesh, usually in the face of a vacancy. This is the same vacancy that I sit in, in my analyst's chair, day after day. How do the others bear this demand? How do they not despair? How do they accept this asymmetrical monetary exchange, something for nothing? How do I?

Sometimes I envy the others. I wonder what they have or imagine they have to offer. What do *they* say? In the face of this burden, what I offer is something of a sham, and I know it. One truth of psychoanalysis is that we cannot really expect help from anyone when it comes down to the brutal realities of life. Whether this has to do with the nature of help or the excess in expectation isn't clear. It may have more to do with the fact that no one ultimately knows. I know all the clichés concerning the curative nature of this nonresponse, this supposedly honest but difficult truth. I'm not certain this isn't simply self-justification. Since we never know if we can help a patient in advance, the more certain we are of our knowledge and the methods of its deployment, the worse the odds become, especially if we are certain about the nature of uncertainty. This uncertain uncertainty regarding help—and not only the nature of help but the possibility of help—is an unshakable burden.

"Revelation," Agamben remarks, "does not mean revelation of the sacredness of a work, but only revelation of its irreparably profane character. . . . The possibility of salvation begins only at this point" (1993, 90.0). Beginning from the irreparable means that those who proclaim the knowledge or means to help, to offer comfort through mutual despair and outrage, are equally impious. For now, everything must wait, even, or especially, when the other cannot. A question of our relationship to knowledge holds center stage. The conversion of the analyst cannot escape the question of the analytic cure, the end that it must conceptualize. At the same time, what comes from any analysis is always yet to be seen. You can only agree to find out together what will change, what might be known, who either of us will be. Symptom-partners,[3] Lacan called the analytic dyad at times. Strange dilemma. Strange urgency and postponement of urgency at once.

This discordance of time that psychoanalysis brings to the surface is so painful. The "maybe" in maybe later, the ever-present "we shall see." A patient rearranged things in her house so that she couldn't give in to a middle-of-the-night anxiety ritual—usually done in the face of intense discomfort and agony felt in her body—this, after quite some time demanding that I tell her what to do. "What is going to happen when I wake up tonight and nothing is there?" She turned her gaze at me expectantly. "I suppose we are about to find out," I said to her before leaving. I found an email in the morning that said: "I woke up. I didn't do anything. I was fine. I went back to bed." I replied to her that what I found funny was how disappointed she sounded. "Well, it's boring," she exclaimed!

In so many of these moments, there I am, groping to find words just empty enough not to allow a patient to pin too much in the future, on the future. I try to hold where we are in order to wait until tomorrow or next week. Maybe they will have a dream or a revelation, *l'esprit de l'escalier*? Just out the door, just shy of expectation, before the moment of forgetting, there is sometimes an encounter. Sometimes this encounter happens by virtue of me, harnessed through the analysis. Sometimes it doesn't seem able to reach the pitch of intensity that is necessary, and I have to sit on my hands. Sometimes a reference to the pain of the present or the past eases the burden between greetings and the long wait ahead. Psychoanalysis in this mode of exchange is plaintive, not palliative. Palliative is a word, it should be noted, that is most often used in relation to the terminally ill.

In the case of my patient, the demand that she wait allowed her finally to say that the ritual was a replacement for boredom, meaning that there was some excitement there that appeared as this nighttime body in agony. My agony is my boredom; my boredom is my agony. Saying all this doesn't tell us much. We don't know that much more than we did before the ritual was allowed to come to a halt. But in creating the conditions in which she confronted herself in her agony, she announced the presence of a desire—however enigmatic, minimal, and couched in the language of negation—that brought into the present some differential force that changed this body in agony ever so slightly. It is the confrontation with a kind of limit that she feels in her body—I was fine. From this, the "I am bored" surfaces. It evokes an intention while the future of the intention must remain open.

Knowledge—even knowledge that might explain the sudden appearance of this boredom or its historical antecedents—seeks to suture this moment, either in the future or through the erasure of this place, this moment of pure address to me. Instead, I mark it—*you seem disappointed*—to which she corrects me: *it's boring*. I could also choose to say nothing. In silence or speech, I am usually trying to understand what it even means to speak to another person with this body and the great burden that it imposes simply because it never works the way it was supposed to. It is never what it is supposed to be. We share the agony of this body and the wait together.

SUPEREGO

I hope you hear in any "supposed to" the problem of knowledge. It hides in the expectation, in a hidden and unquestioned truth. For my patient, it is true that she both expects nothing—this is the force of a long melancholia—and she expects everything—a kind of oral voracity that made its appearance in her body in the form of this middle-of-the-night agony. All of this is as it is. What emerges in her treatment is "the state of things," which is no small feat. Revelation, as Agamben said, is the emergence of something irreparable—what could not have been any other way (1993, 102.2). Even if this opens by constraining the field, it opens without saying *what* is possible. It opens only by announcing possibility as such. "We can have hope only in what is without remedy" (102.2).[4] There is a fascinating moment that I encounter with many patients—just as they reach an opening, the moment is closed down by them asking me anxiously what they should do. The patient demands an answer before they've even heard what they have just said. Such is the force of closure that can come with the desire to know.

Freud, in *Civilization and Its Discontents* (1930), said that he had stopped expecting anything from civilization. It helped him not overvalue what civilization supposedly had to offer; he didn't care if any of it disappeared. Our judgments, he said, follow from our expectations, and they are mostly attempts to support our illusions with arguments. This is how he circumscribes his hope that in the eternal fight Eros might win out against the death drive. Not it must but it might. I admire Freud's stoicism, or realism, which generally feels beyond me. The demand that I be the one supposed to know—when I never wanted to know for another—feels like too much of a burden. This is a burden I bear as a psychoanalyst with some difficulty on most occasions.

Even if I can refuse knowledge, or rather that my being is one of a refusal in relation to knowing, this does not mean that I can free myself from the expectation or the demand coming from another person. I cannot free myself, yet I am free not to know. This duality in the position of the analyst hits me at the kernel of my own refusal, one that I feel in my body daily—"What do I know?" said with a kind of vengeance. This refusal must be refused, the double negation close to the singular and exceptional "no" of the psychoanalyst—not the no of the law, as some would have it, nor the hard no of an imposition of reality against wistfulness but the "no" of this being without remedy, the "no" of knowing there is no other way but still allowing somewhere the "no" of I do not want this. The law is drained but gentle in this emptiness. Wishing can be reopened and started anew.

This constellation that surrounds the question of knowing is one reason the psychoanalytic profession feels impossible *to me*. I must bear the consequences of an always incomplete but necessary conversion in my relation to knowledge. I must refuse an intractable refusal, never overcoming refusal once and for all but never letting it get away with itself entirely. For other analysts, I suspect they have their own reasons for difficulty. Freud, for one, didn't like to be looked at, and in general he seems to have found women irascible and illogical. Their superego, so he claims, is too brittle—as if this wasn't a self-diagnosis.[5]

Never failing to remark on the contradictions of this female superego, Freud said that women were uneducable and loose while at the same time rigidly punitive and susceptible to shame. His imagination is set loose whenever he broaches the feminine figure—a problem with the gaze returning to him through their eyes. The female body, he said, is too easy a source of secondary gain, either in the realm of beauty or as a place to land punishment by feeling pain, being ill, or living in the presentiment of discomfort. Desire, punishment, refusal, and guilt dance endlessly in feminine flesh. Her discomfort is her supposed neurosis. His discomfort with her discomfort *is* his countertransference, a not wanting to know that spills forward into a knowledge that verges on disgust, uniting him—finally—with his hysteric.

For Freud, who knew how to survive over thirty operations on his mouth, this female superego was too wishy-washy—despite the fact he had little Anna there to clean out his wounds.[6] From my perspective, the play of submission and refusal in the feminine superego may not be as decidedly reprehensible as Freud imagines it to be. The conundrums of the superego still sit heavily on psychoanalysts whose post-Freudian inventions, I would wager, converge here—namely, around Freud's countertransference problems.[7] Take Kleinian psychoanalysis and ego psychology, two theories that found their twin solutions: reparation and adaptation.[8] Unconscious guilt is mitigated through a psychic appeal to gratitude and compromise. Gratitude softens pent-up aggression as much as compromise seeks a solution to warring faculties of the mind. Even if these are psychological tendencies, and one can certainly glean their presence in clinical work, I wouldn't rush to judgment that they form some kind of moral ideal.

Reparation and compromise, if they are demanded from the position of the psychoanalyst, quickly collapse into a form of punishment or fantasy of salvation. These solutions are simply a priori on the table. There is nothing to find in analytic work except perhaps the point at which the analyst can levy their cherished opinion, even if it is only the silently held sigh of "ah, finally" or "there you are, I've been waiting." If what is being sought is a solution—certainly to guilt, aggression, and sex—then why wouldn't the possibility of what this looked like be absolutely open? Some mitigation of the superego is necessary in order to maintain neutrality and function as a psychoanalyst, yet the superego is the final lingering conundrum of the psychoanalytic project—a fact that begins to undermine the very ethical foundation of our capacity to work. We still do not know what to say about what happens to a patient's superego at the end of analysis. If no one escapes the relationship to internal commandment, if no one escapes the wish for salvation, perhaps the prototypical hysterical bodily refusal of it is worth further consideration. Considering this symptomatic feminine superego in detail, we might find other, unknown possibilities in the very fact that she continues to search for a way out. If I find trouble in being a psychoanalyst—a kind of stubborn feminine wrestling with demand, especially the imposition of knowledge—there is something more to understand here.

Contrast this hysterical search for a way out with what a priori feels settled in the image of a refined and civilized man or woman, especially when properly rational or compromising or reparative. Imagine all that we can learn from the supposedly female superego: namely, that bodily pain is a way of dealing with the wish for salvation in the face of so little that can be known about the future; that the demand that one assume a position of individual authority, while also bowing to others, she turns into an anxiety run rampant as retaliation; that intergenerational trauma leans on the superego as a way of continually dispensing judgment in order to decide who is bad, who is to blame, who is the culprit, which she takes in too much; and finally that the demand for knowledge touches one deeply, first as an inadequacy and second as a silencing, especially of the vicissitudes of sexuality. This is how I translate Freud's characterization of the female superego as inexorable.

Hysterics are known for the way they keep to a certain kind of refusal. They are creatures of complaint. If complaint is transformed at all, it is perhaps not because the hysteric does not want to complain but because she has lived out how little it works to her advantage, has learned that it brings with it a heap of people with knowledge on offer trying to shut that complaint up. She raises too much in the other the specter of the superego. Nevertheless, what she brings to the table with her complaint is a certain kind of encounter with others, an encounter most are unwilling to face. One might think of Lacan's claim that the hysteric is often cured of everything except her hysteria. One can hear this in the negative, meaning she is a better master than the superego, or one can hear it in the positive sense of cultivating this capacity for an encounter without judgment.

Work with patients has shown me the constant companionship of an extremely intact superego, one that you are never supposed to leave, so it never leaves you alone. This superegoic omnipresence beguiles psychoanalysts, given that we live in a world that almost everyone seems to think of as postmoral. But that is precisely the point. Without external policing, which can function as a relief, an internal force that is inescapable is allowed to rear its ugliest head—something Freud pointed to in the last half of *Civilization and Its Discontents*. The vicissitudes of the superego in the forms of guilt, punishment, and anxiety are rampant. They call upon the analyst as a seer or guide or commanding officer, a call that must be resisted at all costs. The "supposed to" of supposed knowing meets with the "supposed to" in the obscene force of the Panopticon-like superego.[9]

Many tried to find the answer to Freud's bewilderment concerning the phylogenetic heritage of guilt. If it wasn't the collective unconscious written into our DNA to blame, it must be a developmental process where internalization is shaped by caregivers and littered with unconscious fantasies. We can find Lacan joining this conversation but from a completely oblique angle, namely, around the failure of human sexuality pure and simple. Look here! Look at the impasses of the sexual, he seems to want to cajole the analysts. Lacan implores the female analysts in his audience to tell him what they know about sex and the superego, since it was clear to him that they make better analysts—that is, when they are not the worst. Lacan called Anna Freud sinister, sometimes depicted Melanie Klein as omnipotence incarnate, and spoke of women psychoanalysts as forming themselves in the image of the worst primary-school teachers—all is discipline and punishment.

If Freud didn't want to be looked at, Lacan didn't want to be trained or controlled or restrained, especially by women, and forwent seeing Freud because that would mean submitting to another grand dame, the Princess Bonaparte, who happened to be Lacan's analyst's lover. The difference—small, no doubt—between the best and the worst of women as Lacan would define it seems to revolve around a central relationship to the body. A distinct feminine enjoyment is something potentially there as a different tie to the world and others, though when it is missing or clouded over, one might, he felt, do best to run for shelter. She might, if she is lucky, take to castration like a fish in water, since she begins there, Lacan said of women. Women at times like fish.

While Freud is the unmoved mover—he was never analyzed—Lacan, on the other hand, seems to have disavowed his analysis in its entirety as some sort of process of normalization, in other words, as a superegoic endeavor. This shouldn't mean that Lacan didn't have an experience of analysis despite his analyst. After everything that happened to Lacan, he still wrote rather touching letters to Löwenstein attesting to what he had received from the analysis and how it helped him in his trials with the psychoanalytic institution. "I dream of that kind of faith which carries me now beyond all this, which almost makes me forget it," Lacan writes to Löwenstein in a sentence of the strangest tenses ([1973] 1990, 64).

By "all this," he meant the institution of psychoanalysis. By "beyond," he meant the experience he had of psychoanalysis with Löwenstein, which he says he had only recently begun to understand. It has made him more certain of "his fate and his destiny" (64). From the *this* of the psychoanalytic institution to another *this*, one's destiny, Lacan makes an appeal to his former analyst. At the very end of the letter to Löwenstein, he says he would like to offer him some freedom—not to add what he has said to a dossier (though sadly, I think Löwenstein did)—but instead to find the freedom that their special relationship accords them and to hear the testimony that Lacan gives, without which history could not have been written. He asks Löwenstein to be this fish, to take to the water in the same way Lacan was only beginning to learn to—the special freedom that psychoanalysis offers where you can swim like women.

Lacan was asking for a psychoanalytic institution that mirrored this special freedom, that worked in accordance with a subversion of the superego, and that could hold a respect for all that it takes to meet one's destiny. Destiny in Lacan, especially in this earlier period, acts as a counterforce to a superego that always tries to delay the future, especially the future in the guise of fulfillment. We can locate here a strange oxymoron in what it means to be a psychoanalyst: one is never free of the onslaught of demands coming from a patient, their judgment or helplessness, yet one is free not to know, free to proceed into the future, free to be this fish, drop all superegoic responses to demand, in oneself and from others. This is the limited, though difficult, freedom granted by psychoanalysis.

If we assume that every analyst has to wrestle with some constellation of superegoic forces, then no psychoanalyst will ever live in some hallowed ground of *having been analyzed*. What we can know intimately about the conundrum is what the analyst can do. Perhaps this is why Lacan stresses that the analyst is simply the one who knows how to take up a certain position—what we might call the conversion of the analyst—in the face of what is impossible. This is also why Lacan asks the analyst to rest against one of the clearest points of opposition in Freud to the superego, namely, the body and the drive—to venerate their structural refusal.[10]

In moving from analysand to psychoanalyst, from couch to chair, questions remain. What do you take with you? What do you leave behind? What is transformed in this movement from one place to the other that allows the analyst to become an analyst? What must the analyst know, when all is said and done? What part does their being play, in its fish and flesh, in being a psychoanalyst? What is this conversion of the analyst-patient to the analyst proper? This last question feels particularly important if one is gripped by the shimmering lights of hysteria—blinding body, all pain, all symptomatic contortions of ignorance and the glory of a world that arrives from nowhere. The silent, still, contained, unknowing position of the analyst does not necessarily seem the obvious vocation. Lacan wanted to give psychoanalysts an out, a way to slip out the back door—to do it on tiptoe—even if they were the ones who snuck in in the first place. It isn't clear, he says, that having undergone an analysis should produce the desire to be an analyst at all.

Perhaps we might imagine that it would be quite to the contrary: that having unraveled all this matter out, the pain of this psychical work would allow one to leave once and for all; that the refusal could become absolute—could be the very refusal of psychoanalysis. For the obstinate Lacan, this might even be better proof of the analyst-patient's conversion. "Why are any of you here?" Lacan sometimes questioned his audience, begging them to explain what they found in their analysis that might inform this desire that he called "un-normal" or "a-normal," emphasizing the negative, the loss of any point of normality, and the attachment of the analyst to a special point on the body—the psychoanalytic soma-object of desire—that he indicates with the letter *a*.

This statement is more than a statement against the normal, though it is that too. Lacan is looking for the horizon beyond anything natural or supposedly human. The permanent pressure of drive life that characterizes soma and what it means to have a sexual body—this driven momentum—Lacan considered inhuman, as a machinelike dimension of the body whose constant movement and pressure begs for the conversion of energy. Psychoanalysis cultivates this plea for conversion that it does not answer. Why, one might ask, would anyone willingly suffer—especially when we are not all advocates of masochism—this embarrassing, painful position as a psychoanalyst, a name that ironically has engendered the most bitter of professional wars? "Say something about why you do not make a hasty exit! Tell me what passes for the desire to be a psychoanalyst!" Lacan berates his listeners.

The desire of the analyst, Lacan claims, must be carried by the drive. In being able to pass through a certain threshold of tension, there is an alteration in the structure or grip of the superego. This is Lacan's challenge to reparation or adaptation or any mitigated idealism or form of adjustment as the normalizing goal of psychoanalysis. The desire of the analyst is for the continuation of psychoanalysis to whatever end, not for any particular end. What kind of desire is this? Is it monstrously inhuman, ethical, or somehow both? How far must one go to find the edge that dissolves everything?

The portrait that Lacan paints of the "other side" of the threshold isn't some moral paradise: The body is still a burden on being, the absolute separation of truth from knowledge will remain, the encounter with the abyss of human illusion is terrifying and unending, and in our private relationship with death we can expect help from no one. Psychoanalysis leads to something like an encounter with this irreparable ground, this hopeless hope, where the work—like mourning—continues to be painful. Freud always said psychical work of this nature was equivalent to actual physical pain. It isn't a metaphor. Unbinding, as a work of the death drive, is an absolutely material pain. It is a bodily disordering, a material disorder. But it is the material necessary for becoming a psychoanalyst. This is the conversion disorder at the heart of the act of becoming an analyst.

CONVERSION DISORDER

Conversion disorder is a late-nineteenth-century term fastened to hysteria, which it eclipses when hysteria disappears in the 1980s from psychiatry all together. Conversion remains—more ambiguous than hysteria and certainly more gender neutral. It is less arduous of a term than "conversion hysteria" and much emptier in appearance than just "hysteria," which evokes too many images of mad women—*les hystériques*. Conversion is found lumped under the heading of the somatoform disorders, congruent with psychosomatic illness, or under a new heading: functional neurological symptom disorder, as if general concerns with soma are irrelevant.

I am happy to greet the word "form" in all of this, if not the conjoined terms psyche-soma or even the word functional—the word lingers in order to convey the constancy of dysfunction, the order always hoped for in disorder. Conversion is also linked to the dissociative disorders. All these terms taken together form a strange series that runs between conversion, hysteria, soma, form, function, dissociation, and splitting, retaining the traces and tracks of history even as the overt aim was to erase a presence of the history of conversion as tied to Freud, starting with having the word "hysteria" ousted from the psychiatric bible. The irony is that hysteria preceded Freud from the Greeks to Janet and Charcot[11] whereas conversion was a term uniquely deployed by Freud, which—as we will see—underlies much of his theoretical work, perhaps even more than the esteemed *hysteria*.

The turning of the tides from conversion to hysteria and back seems to speak to something that insists—certainly on the level of the body—but that is always more than just that: psyche-soma, soma-form, function-form, split soma, divided psyche. Whatever this consistent reference to the body is meant to imply, it is linked to the history of medicine and psychiatry. It is a concept that always hovers on a border and is ripe for this constellating force. This is close to the way Freud worked with his notion of the drive, something he always called a limit concept and a concept on the limit between the psychic and somatic.[12] It pleases me that this is so despite the persistent outcry of psychoanalysts against the disappearance of the term "hysteria." Why? What is the dependence on terminology?

We might welcome this word *conversion*, coined in any case by Freud. It is pure psychoanalytic nomenclature, grounded in Freud's model of the psyche from his early neurological research. The transfer of energy from one sphere of the mind to another or from one material form to another is conversion. The term "conversion" interrupts the quest of psychiatry, evoked as both the thing itself *and* a strange remainder or surplus in relation to it. The contemporary moment wants to retain this word *conversion*, in a world that has dispensed with psychoanalysis while remaining rife with problems circling around religious, economic, and political violence, each one tied to questions of—if not longings for—conversion, transformation, total change. The points where the body speaks of its insoluble pains turn around the place where this word takes hold: religious conversion, the problems of fundamentalism, the impotent attempts to extract politics from theology, a biopolitical era whose force of regulation touches us all on a bodily level, reaching into every crevice, like the endless movements of currency, economic conversions on small and large scales, against the background of unthinkable economic disparity and inequality.

Like a hidden abyss, mysterious diseases travel along the fault lines of culture—a culture that promises sheer spectacle when it isn't promising future disaster. Maybe conversion will tell us why any of us carry on, why bodily disorder and the promise of transformation—body and soul—slip into every realm of life. What remains? What is possible? What kind of conversion may be hoped for? I want to know for myself psychoanalysis as conversion disorder—as the disorder of conversion—in order to live with what is rightfully called the impossible profession. I would like to understand something more about this vocational calling, this conversion our profession depends upon without ever being able to theorize it fully. I would like to know something more about this strange choice of profession.

A day doesn't go by where I don't find myself imagining the many other ways of being than that of a psychoanalyst, a life that might exclude me from the position of having to know very much at all so that I can be in my body in a different way—not in this chair, not burdened by an unfulfillable demand, caught somewhere between voice and ear. Wouldn't it be lovely to be a stenographer, who only knows with her fingers, or a waitress knowing with her body, eyes closed, how to navigate a crowded room, arms full of what is meant to satiate, delivered as ordered. Where is conversion in this psychopathology of everyday life? Where is it confined when an occupation can be kept apart from any need for transformation? What is a vocation if I need not transform a thing? Devotion without vocation? Transformation without devotion?

I can also imagine being a housewife, with her expectable though by no means less unbearable pain. The pain of a housewife in the time of feminism. To live in that contradiction—a bourgeois contradiction—holding fast at the beginning of psychoanalysis and all of its bored women patients. I see her now as she throws herself into the daily routine—a driver, a babysitter, a house manager, an escort, or a companion. The emptier the better, the fuller, the greater the threat of symptomatic pains that write themselves on her flesh: strange autoimmune diseases; obscure aches; a litany of possible diseases; with medications on offer, some taken; and the infinite number of people at your disposal that you can pay to treat weary flesh. A body between the cracks. Please touch me. Tell me where it hurts. With these healers of various sorts, she is given a place to know herself in some other way, to have herself again, as a body in pain but attended to by others.

We are still living in the nineteenth century. Hydrotherapy and sanatoriums have other names, including the recourse to seaside vacation or energy work or massage. On the less privileged end, it is somewhat the same as it was; the barbaric institutions of psychiatric facilities or prison are tempting,[13] a solution to an inequitable and counterproductive fight for protection and stability. All of these are places where one can hide for a time from the demands of efficiency and productivity leveled at one's body. The sanatoriums were traded for family life, a prison for a prison. The decision is made on the basis of a distinct claim made by a supposedly sick body or criminal conscience. The body has its ways of disordering one prison and erecting others. All wind their way toward punishment and the ad hoc demands of guilt.

The superego is caught in the vicissitudes of compliance and defiance, while the quest for what would feel productive, and so free from guilt, is trapped in questions of utility, pacification, and security. There is nothing less productive than a body that always makes a break for it; it does what it likes. We can, if we wish, give ourselves over to the pathos of fascination with the grace of athleticism and the tragedy of its rapid decline: the fear of aging, not of dying. Perhaps we might keep vigilance through hypochondria, the bastard child of conversion disorder. For the rest of us, without the energy or time for this level of maintenance, the body will not easily submit to the demand for a seamless everyday life, the routines of work and relaxation doled out in expectable rhythms, even when those become the sixty-hour work week or the doldrums of the search for employment. Life degrades to an impossible search for the point of utmost order, the pure stasis of an order that can never be kept.

Stasis, we might remember, is Greek for civil war. Stasis is a breakdown in an economy or system of exchange that requires openings at the border between the inside and outside. Stasis acts as tinder for the fire of interior strife. Civil war for the Greeks is always about to erupt and is another name for conversion disorder. This errant body is supposed to be tamed and turned toward the aims of civilization, and we, unable to fulfill this task, are left with discontent, malaise, and nausea as iterations of stasis. To add insult to injury, one often feels guilty for being so ill at ease, while this body gone rogue can offer itself as an easy host to this guilt. Psychoanalysts used to call this "secondary gain." How?

What gain, when this is simply the condition of living together, where universal discontent means the neurotic baseline of a sick body that we are all supposed to figure out how to live with? It feels to me more like secondary pain. At the extreme end, we land on the guilty self-attack of a depressive whose illness renders their body simply vegetative, a-rhythmic, unemployable. Freud likened the effects of depression on libido to a siphon with no container. One's body as the source of depletion, with no bottom or zero point, *is* pure pain; it is the paradox of a container that ceases to function as a container and nevertheless has no outside. No gain but this tradeoff: one living hell, external, for another, internal. At least one's internal hell can be of one's own making. At least, in this conversion disorder, there is something of a conversion that one might call *mine*. My sickness, my pain.

Conversion comes from the Latin *convertere*, which means to turn around, or altogether turn, seeming to speak to the minimal difference between repetition, what keeps turning and turning, and change, what is overturned. Conversion disorder seems to carry with it the absolutely singular, one's particular conversion, while keeping this tied to what is universal, namely, what is our disorder, all together. Everything or nothing will be overturned. Even when conversion degrades from the religious to the material, from spirit, *Geist*, to the object—the symptom of all symptoms, according to Marx, is the conversion of labor to currency—you still retain something of the all-together turning evoked by the word. One can imagine here the infinite charting of currency across the world like temperamental streaks of light on a sky that fills all nights. Economically, we turn all together, like today's global markets.

Conversion, many have said, arises only with Judeo-Christian religion or religion insofar as it involves an experience of conversion and the desire to convert. Various pagan religions or cults were more ecumenical, bound to location and culture, changing and evolving with time, introducing new deities, rites, and customs, sometimes integrating or assimilating other religions when war brought them into contact. A. D. Nock in his classic study *Conversion* writes, "by conversion we mean the reorientation of the soul of an individual, his deliberate turning from indifference or from an earlier form of piety to another, a turning which implies a consciousness that great change is involved, that the old was wrong and the new is right" (1933, 7).

Nock, following Nietzsche's *On the Genealogy of Morals*, aims to demonstrate that prophetic religions and philosophy, opposed to paganism up to the time of Alexander, worked by conversion. They used intellectual and emotional conviction in the struggle of what is right against what is evil, but they made this conviction available to all, not just the wealthy or literate. Nock argues that the pagan tradition operated according to adhesion or assimilation—namely, taking everything in that can be used for the interests of empire. The prophetic religions and philosophies, while narrower, were more democratic.

While Nock seems to want to discredit religions of conversion for their moral certainty, he nevertheless paints another portrait, one where conversion is the act whereby something latent meets with a catalyst: "it is not a conversion from indifference; it is a progress in a continuous line; it is like a chemical process in which the addition of a catalytic agent produces a reaction for which all the elements were already present" (266). The prophet is someone who knows the hothouse in which he lives, knows how to "fuse into a white heat" the combustible material that is there to express and "to appear to meet the half-formed prayers" of his contemporaries (266). In other words, the prophet is someone who understands how to listen to the prayers of the present. In this picture of conversion, what is right and what is wrong is less at the center than this process of combustion that changes everything for a person, that turns their soul inside out and reorients them by virtue of something speaking to their hidden desires and fears. The older religions, from paganism to Mithraism and Gnosticism, lost the battle when they fell out of touch with their time and assumed that what was was enough.

Nock ends his book by saying that this groping for an ultimate reality leaves something missing, as must have been the case for all those groping. To study history is to study ruins. Yet what is finally revealed is the obscure, precisely as obscure, at the center of a prayer. Conversion is a confrontation with what will always remain veiled; it is a practice that kneels before the ineffable and nonetheless, touching this point, changes something. Where Nock imagines his text to fail, in fact, is where it reveals its truth. Conversion is not so different from the earlier religions that bore witness to the obscure power of the gods in everyday life, which required neither conversion nor belief because the world around was felt to be enchanted. What conversion does differently, however, is to meet a growing need to speak about matters of disenchantment, disappointment, and ennui. Is conversion simply a reenchantment that comes with a prophetic encounter? How do we understand this malaise so long before this disenchantment, which is usually associated with modernity? It is here, with this disenchantment that reaches back thousands of years, that I would like to place psychoanalytic conversion next to religious conversion.

ADVENT OF THE ANALYST

Why become a psychoanalyst? Lacan was never satisfied with the answers he was given by his colleagues. He then decided to labor over another question—what is psychoanalysis? Might we find an answer to his other question here? In his 1971–1972 seminar, *The Knowledge of the*

Psychoanalyst, he states, "it is the mapping out of what is understood as obscure, of what is obscured in understanding because of a signifier which marked a point of the body" (98). A point of the body, not a point on the body—an important distinction because even while the point is marked as a clash between word and flesh, it is *of* the body, meaning it is already body.

The signifier has its own materiality such that this is a point of contact, flesh with flesh. It is precisely this materiality that remains obscure in understanding, which persists as *the* challenge to knowledge. The signifier is on the side of the body: "what speaks . . . is what enjoys itself as a body" (98). At other times, Lacan delineates this simply as the field of the sexual, and Freud, it must be remembered, persists with the equation between body and sexuality. Analysis reproduces this point, this moment where flesh divides the flesh—and how could this not be sexual?—in order to attest to what is obscure in life. It materializes and crystallizes the sexual.

Everyone, Lacan says, oddly enough, agrees on this. In this reproduction, the analyst is in the same position as the parent who produced the trauma, the parent whose work is to organize the bodies of their children with his or her own, always calling upon his or her sexual life and sexual history. This, he says again with great assurance, is what we call transference. A peculiar set of remarks, especially insofar as he imagines all analysts agree upon this, as if agreement was common or even possible between analysts, especially with regard to such enigmatic moments, no less the place of sexuality. This obsession with origins in psychoanalysis, the attempt to pinpoint something so primary in the strange life of the human being, is best thought of in structural terms. Otherwise, at least for Lacan, we lapse into normative developmental fictions. We need to understand the advent of the body as sexual and signifiable.

This points to a question not just about the origins of the subject but about the analyst's body in analysis as well. While much of what one might hear about "Lacanian" analysts is their fidelity to language, or to the "desire of the analyst" for psychoanalysis, or their role as provocateur, dummy, death's head in the bridge game or chess match of psychoanalysis, there are many points in which all this slips away, where what analysis is for Lacan is something that takes place in and through the psychoanalyst's body. These latter remarks may be more uncomfortable than the other images of a virtuoso at work, even more uncomfortable than when these images are reduced to the skillful deployment of the silent dummy or the court jester. What can a psychoanalyst do with their body for another? A body that more than anything is to remain silent, still, and seated? Still, in order to open one's ear?

Lacan gave the reply to the question "what is psychoanalysis?" at the Sainte-Anne Hospital, where his lectures began and where he formed himself as a psychoanalyst. Returning to Sainte-Anne after many years, he wonders what he's come back to tell. What he ends up saying to the new cadre of psychiatrists is that the psychoanalyst is not very free in the arrangement of psychoanalysis—an odd message perhaps referring to his own history. He returned to Sainte-Anne in order to say something in the place where he discovered what it meant to be a psychoanalyst. He says that the analyst has to reawaken this mark of the body that is the point of disorder, not to adapt this disorder to the order of the day, nor to make reparations to the souls who we believe were the cause of its pain, but rather in the name of spreading this disorder, converting a piece of reality into it.

"The difference," says Lacan, "is that the psychoanalyst, from his position reproduces the neurosis[,] and the traumatic parent for his part produces it innocently" (99). The analyst *reproduces*—causes to repeat—this point, this bodily event that shapes our being. Lacan calls this the signifier in its efflorescence. A place where something takes root in us—constellating our enjoyment and pain, organizing the surface of the body around a moment out of joint—that we must repeat. Repeat, in order to complete it. Forcing it to join with itself, flesh with flesh. There is something half done in us. Repeat it! All the way this time, however painful, conjuring everything in its wake in order to then, and only then, simplify it, crystallize it. In other words, to convert it. Oddly enough, it turns out that what is being converted has very little to do with a subject, self, or identity.

We must evoke the formal brilliance of an originary body, provoking and repeating this body through the relationship between patient and doctor. This is done in order to return this *whatever-it-is* to our patients, showing the luminous somatoform stamp that inhabits desire. Returning it, returning to it, drains some of the attachment to suffering—in particular in relation to so many half-repetitions caught in the wrappings of meaning, history, fantasy, where it always tends to asphyxiate. The conversion of the patient in analysis takes place through repeating in his or her body the mark of its disorder. The sick body is made into an analytic body through the analyst, who holds open a space for work.

"It must give you the shivers, what I am saying!?" Lacan chides his audience. "It is from the phantasy of the psychoanalyst, namely, from what is most opaque, most closed, most autistic in his word, that there comes the shock by which the word is unfrozen in the analysand" (1967–1968, 195–96). Later, Lacan will call this process a "corporeal deduction." This corporeal process makes the analyst one's own. This is not a metaphorical process! The analyst is not *like* one's mother, or one's mother's breast, or breast milk—the analyst *is* these things, made into them by the patient, in order finally not to be them. The ultimate concreteness: the analyst is a breast. But also for Lacan, the most original form of identification: I am the object. "The hysteric reaches the goal immediately. The Freud she is kissing is the object. Everyone knows this is what a hysteric needs when coming out of hypnosis. Things are in a certain way, as one might say, cleared away" (196). Contra so much thought on the supposed difference between the concrete thing and metaphorical language, between thing and word representation, here we aim—oddly—against the structures of meaning and metaphor.

If Lacan generally eschews knowledge given as directive, in this moment where he returns to the Hospital Sainte-Anne, he provides the analysts with the clearest of maps: all of this "is a matter of knowing what exists" (1971–1972, 132). It is a matter of what is real. This is what the psychoanalysis stages an encounter with, the paradox being that for Lacan what is real always escapes knowledge. This obscure point of the body escapes in order to mark something in the future, to be conjured by this doctor—this is what there is. Freud says to Fliess in a letter from 1899, "What happened in earliest childhood?" The answer: "Nothing, but the germ of a sexual impulse existed" (1985, 338). The ambiguity holds in

German: nothing but the germ of a sexual impulse, nothing but also the germ of a sexual impulse.

In a strange optics of time, what failed to happen in the past, by virtue of what did, returns in the present to clear out the future, like a dream's day residue of frustrated wishes returning in order to construct the most indelible desires. This is what we cannot see—the object that I am, the contingencies, the traumas, what cast us aside. Agamben configures the structure philosophically: "it does not will to repeat the past in order to consent to what has been, transforming 'so it was' into 'so I willed it to be.' On the contrary, it wills to let it go, to free itself from it, in order to gain access beyond, or on this side of the past to what has never been, to what was never willed. Only at this point is the unlived past revealed for what it was: contemporary with the present" (2009, 103). This unlived past is brought to life in the analyst's body, history becoming seamless with the present through the analytic dyad. The advent of the analyst happens in this strange reawakening of the patient's body in ours. If this is true, I'm surprised analysts aren't more resistant to psychoanalysis, or, to turn this around, perhaps this is why they are, why psychoanalysis is dying. Who would want to make themselves the vessel for so many others in this way? To have them repeat their pain and unlived life in your flesh?

I DON'T WANT TO BE A PSYCHOANALYST

After a decade in private practice, after hours and hours of listening to patients—mostly women, it must be said—and without a single one whom I wouldn't describe as touching the realm of so-called conversion disorder, I fell on an impossible desire to write a book about the body as it makes its appearance to me in sessions—the singular stamp of a patient's body in their dream life, sexual fantasies, modes of enjoyment, ways of speaking, gestural habits, and aesthetic wrappings. A book looking at the repetitive insistence of their body in its singularity and the way it erupts in analysis at critical moments—an impossible intimacy that I am granted, that I feel only I am granted (rightly or wrongly) by virtue of holding this seat as their analyst.

This body was the one thing that could carry both patient and analyst across the most difficult moments, and this meant having to lean into sexuality. I look for it, and I listen for it, and nothing has proven a better guide than these tracks of what we never have or, to turn it around, what we may only have. To show this body as the cosmos that Freud returned to us—a star map—not just for the analyst, who knows only too much about the body (to the point that nothing can be said), but also for the patient, who isn't required to know a thing. Patients—and you should note here the trace of envy—simply find their way, enter back into the everyday. We have to carry on.

With this nonknowledge, this map held at the threshold of inside and outside, I imagined this book in the form of a *corps morcelé*, the evocation of the body in bits and pieces like a liturgy in reverse, not body as word but word become body. The book would serve as a prayer in the direction of this body, or the prayer as body par excellence. A series of luminous fragments of analysis shown as bound to something so physical, material. And how wonderful all of these parts are: eyes, hands, anus, mouth, breasts, clitoris, vagina, phallus, feet, nose, ears, neck, back. Each one its own chapter. Each one an end in itself.

> *In my dream I was watching them waltz, which became more and more erotic. I didn't know what they were doing. I was feeling more and more confused. Are they? Anticipation and confusion mixed into the strangest feeling, anxiety on the cusp of the orgasmic. And then he put his finger in her ass, and I thought to myself, now I know they are fucking! Why does the ass tell me something with so much certainty, I ask in this office everyday. Why is it the source where my anxiety can appear and disappear? I know you think it's because I want to do everything back to front.*

> *I had a dream about* The King and I, *except it was spelled:* The King and Eye. *It's the sentence for my entire analysis. This belief in being able to*

see 360 degrees, a massive eyeball. It is why I can't help thinking I will be shot by a sniper when I run below an underpass; why I have this fantasy that I can see everything, know everything, Google everything. I downloaded the app Freedom the other day, amused by the name—it shuts down the internet. I started to think the other day that it's not only the anxiety of influence; it's the ecstasy of influence, also.

I had a feeling like there were snakes in the wall. All bunched up in there together. I could hear the rustling of their skin as they wrestled with one another. A horrible sound. Or was it a feeling? It is my body, this soundfeeling. It is the exquisite agony of anxiety in my skin. Writhing, rustling, wrestling, restless. I don't know if it is this place of contact—skin—this living barrier between myself and everything else or the feeling of being too close in spite of a limit. I want to be by myself. Those snakes follow me into this prison that I erected for my own safety.

When I reached to grab my checkbook this morning to pay you, my new sex toy was there, and I thought I can't tell her about this. Why? Because it's like a part of my body that I had to go find. And it's so hard to reconcile giving so much power to something outside of you, even if it feels like it is you. I have this joke about the uncanny valley where you can go to find all these things that are human and inhuman at once, this treasure trove of all the pieces of myself that I have lost. I said to my father the other day, don't make a mountain out of this. He doesn't know that I live in this valley, which I think of as my depression. But this sex toy feels like the first time I have taken something out of there into real life, and I guess it's what I paid you for.

I was throwing up, and I wanted to blame you, like you did this to me, it was all your fault, and then at the same time it felt good, felt good to eat and then to get rid of all of it, and I thought about you holding my hair, waiting patiently. I can't think because I'm hungry, and I'm hungry because I can't think. Or, if I was going to put it another way, I have always just needed to die. I just don't know what that means yet. I feel like you could tell me, and you won't. Or would, if it wasn't for the fact that I'm so hungry, and I don't know how to stop it, and all I do is come in here and tell you that. I can't stand anymore, I feel like those people being jostled on the subway. All my bones are breaking. What can't you stand? I can't stand on the ground, I told you this . . . My body. But I guess what I really can't stand is my body.

I can feel the hormones as they are depleting, as if my muscles become softer, and something even happens to the shape of my face. I feel this softness around the left side of my abdomen. I was examining my testicles the other day and I think I can see the place they are injured. Every time I masturbate I check to see the extent of the damage. I can't get an erection anymore. None of the doctors want to deal with me, but I know I have a real problem. It is in my body. And I begin to feel more and more like a woman, as if my male hormones are drained, and I have this feeling like I'm turning into this little bitch, this moaning whore. I can't think after that. You don't believe me. That I feel this sick. That my brain shuts down. You think it's in my mind. Let me tell you, I'm not the only one obsessed with hormones. The whole world is.

My shoulders are in pain and my neck is tight after all these surgeries from fighting. I always thought it was strength, and I'm only now realizing it's about flexibility at the point where I can barely move anymore. I guess the joke is on me, but I don't want to take this any further than it being a joke, because then the physical is metaphysical, and you know I can't stand that. I'm not into hocus-pocus. I keep it in the writing, Doc, where I'm comfortable with metaphor or even magic because it's squarely a fiction. If it blurs too much in reality, I get very uncomfortable. So let's just say I had a lesson to learn about what it takes to fight, and I got the values wrong.

That phrase keeps coming back, ashes in my mouth. It's the only thing that feels true to say. I read everything online about mourning, and the stages, and what is helpful, and who. People come and they say the things that people say, but what I can't say back, and what no one wants to hear, and what is the only true thing, is that it is ashes in my mouth, and then I want to scream at them about the moment when I knew he was going to die, how you feel it on the inside, and nothing will ever be the same. There was the moment before and the moment after and all of it I know inside my mouth.

I have to walk sometimes for a very long time. Something in me begins to stiffen and close. It has something to do with judgment, as if it creeps over my whole body and drags even thinking to a standstill. It's funny because writing and painting are the only things that save me from this feeling, but I can't do them all day long, so at some point I have to leave the house because if I stay I'll read things on the internet, like the news, and the judgment begins to creep in that way. I'm reading and a strange kind of enjoyment in judging what is before my eyes is suddenly there, you can't help but go there, and the inevitable next question will be—who do you think you are? As if you are any better? The way this question boomerangs back, it hits you on the inside and everything stiffens. All I can do is try to wake up new.

I could describe this pain like a phantom limb; it just feels like even when it's not there, it is still there, or the attachment to it is there, like the raised red scar of an old wound that you continually touch and never seems to heal. When I say this to you I want to know if you will fix me, if this means that I'm broken, and at the same time I'm afraid of this idea, because the pain is there for a reason, it commemorates something, it is about what is wrong, and isn't it wrong to believe that something isn't wrong and to not have that as a constant presence in your life, defining who you are—I am this set of scars, this phantom pain.

I could go on with more examples, with many of my other patients. These stories are all body—startlingly so—forming a specifically demarcated point in an analysis. It is a body that addresses another from some other place; nothing here belongs either to the analyst or the patient alone.

This body and whatever "I" the patient can lay claim to condense such that this whatever-it-is—I as subject, I as object, body, sex—presents itself to the analysis. Writing this writing of the body as it unfolds, it felt important to evoke this process in its absolute materiality, its pulsating presence, the undulating surface that carries these analyses along. This sentence is my entire analysis. This sentence is my body. Each sentence writes Freud's *Three Essays on the Theory of Sexuality*, showing us the lifecycle as bound to the stamp of the body in the staccato, unruly rhythms of sexuality.

To what end? To mark something in the past? To grasp a now that is constantly in the process of being deferred? To grind to a halt the machine that is trying to force this body into one pathway, one measure, one reality—a reality that Lacan says is decidedly not real. The origin of the subject linked to the end of analysis becomes a tale told through a patient's body! This, I realized, is a book that simply cannot be written. It is too intimate to reveal the details of a patient's analysis in the way I imagine it must be done.

Flesh redividing flesh, even if done in order to show the process by which a psychoanalytic cure takes place, is the secret of every psychoanalysis. This would be too objectifying in the manner and detail I had imagined it should be done. Potentially, this might be where Freud's case studies caused so much trouble for his patients. I think it is the revelations of these bodily secrets by Freud, both what was wrong and what was right in them, that continued to affect Little Hans, Dora, and the Wolf Man deeply—from fingers touching belts and men touching back, to talk of widdlers and bathroom scenes with mother, to the persistence of a primal-scene fantasy and the way a body can lose control, again and again and again. Hans and Dora only spoke with great hatred for psychoanalysis and their experience with it, while the Wolf Man ended up soldered to it, like some kind of charge of the psychoanalytic institution, renouncing his own name for the one Freud gave him.

To live with my impossible choice of profession, I found myself with the impossible-to-write book—the book that must never cease not to be written. It is at that point, with this attempted solution to the difficulty of enduring a work that on any day is too much to bear, that my body gave out on me. Little aches and pains, larger ones that made their way into a general disordering—nothing was working the way it was supposed to. Like Freud returning from vacation, "my mood, critical faculties, subsidiary ideas—in short, all mental accessories—have been buried under an avalanche of patients" (1985, 330). What other conversion was necessary? What had escaped me in my work as an analyst?

These new symptoms, which could only be given the heading of conversion disorder, felt like a pact with my patients. I did, it is true, on occasion try on their symptoms—unclear how we would both find our way out of this symptomatic labyrinth. We were in it together. Perhaps these symptoms marked a promise held to this book that I could not write where the question of conversion, this body as it appears in a treatment, was something that I could communicate to no one. At the very least, I could console myself—all of this would never amount to the knowledge I never wanted it to be. It would remain unwritten—even when it had written itself.

But one still has to live with all this conversion, this disorder of conversion that is my impossible profession. Is this what I came to find? What it means to live with a body for all its contortions, both brilliant and symptomatic? An impossible sexuality? What am I entitled to say or do as psychoanalyst? The book—as I'm sure has already become clear to you, though it wasn't clear to me for a very long time—would not be about the patient's body. It would have to be about mine: the conversion disorder of the psychoanalyst.

II

MUSIC OF THE FUTURE

Why the formation of symptoms in conversion hysteria should be such a peculiarly obscure thing I cannot tell; but the fact affords us a good reason for quitting such an unproductive field of enquiry without delay.

—SIGMUND FREUD, *INHIBITIONS, SYMPTOMS, AND ANXIETY*

MUSIC OF THE FUTURE

To speak about conversion, we have to return to Freud and Breuer's *Studies in Hysteria* ([1895] 1995) and read the term forward, moving closer to the peculiar and singular place of the body in the construction of the Freudian psyche. "I have a sounding board in my abdomen . . . if anything happens, it starts up my old pain," said a woman to Breuer (204). While hysterical conversion was mostly a female problem (the book consists of five cases, all women), in the section devoted to this diagnosis, Breuer is quick to evoke the figure of a man:

> All degrees of affective excitability are to be found between, on the one hand, the ideal (which is rarely met with today) of a man who is absolutely free from "nerves," whose heart-action remains constant in every situation and is only affected by the particular work it has to perform, the man who has a good appetite and digestion, whatever danger he is in—between a man of this kind and, on the other hand, a "nervous" man who has palpitations and diarrhoea on the smallest provocation.
>
> (203)

The scarce masculine ideal, absolutely free and without "nerves," is opposed to the nervous woman with the sounding board in her abdomen that can revive any old pain. It is the electrified, nerve-ridden body of the hysterical woman that gives the ideal—the unprovoked man—and at the same time completely undermines it. He is rarely met with today. But yesterday? And then what is she?

Only thirty-some-odd pages later, Freud takes over—as he often does—this hysteric's imagery as his own. Through her words, Freud lays the foundation for the existence of "unconscious ideas" and the "splitting" of the mind on the basis of her speaking about her body. It is not the masculine that proves universal but his failed other half, woman, that gives to Breuer and Freud a new model of the relationship between mind and body. Freud writes:

The impressionability of hysterical patients is indeed to a large extent determined simply by their innate excitability; but the lively affects into which they are thrown by relatively trivial causes become more intelligible if we reflect that the "split-off" mind acts like a sounding-board to the note of a tuning fork. Any event that provoked unconscious memories liberates the whole affective force of these ideas that have not undergone a wearing-away, and the affect that is called up is then quite out of proportion to any that would have arisen in the conscious mind alone.

(237–38)

The apparent spontaneity that defines conversion symptoms also defines the women in question. Their bodies and personalities are described in concert: lively, restless, craving sensations and mental stimulation, intolerant of monotony or boredom, sexually excitable, awakened, sometimes infantile (kicking and thrashing about), suggestible, volatile, and whose force of resistance could swing from excessive and rigidly defensive to seemingly weak and utterly permeable. This unity of soma-psyche in conversion hysterics provides Freud, paradoxically, with a model of the disunity of the human mind. Or perhaps better, this logical ordering of their disorder provides Freud with a similar psychological theory concerning the logic of the unconscious.

In hysteria, nothing is subject to the so-called natural processes of erosion: wearing away, draining, leveling, and emptying out. The whole affective force is preserved. The sounding board remains a sounding board, while the question of proportion (out of proportion or in concert with whatever supposed reality) remains a value judgment whose ideal—namely, what's real—is always just out of reach. The goal of psychotherapy, interestingly enough, is not a removal of the pathogenic but a new state altogether. In the greatest of tautologies in psychoanalysis, conversion must be subject to conversion.

This is why Freud must abandon the cathartic aim, the difference between catharsis and conversion being the difference between momentary relief and radical change. Freud famously concludes this early work by saying that patients have made the following objections to him in the course of their analyses: "Why, you tell me yourself that my illness is probably connected with my circumstances and events in my life. You cannot alter these in any way. How do you propose to help me then?" To which he replied, "No doubt fate would find it easier than I do to relieve you of your illness. But you will not be able to convince yourself that much will be gained if we succeed in transforming your hysterical misery into common unhappiness. With a mental life that has been restored to health you will be better armed against that unhappiness" (305). In the case of catharsis, the patient experienced momentary relief, which is a great help in cases of extreme tension but whose effects seemed not to last. The questions remain: What must be altered? What is this transformation or conversion of hysterical misery? What in conversion arms one against unhappiness?

In this little dialogue, the patient knows that the doctor cannot alter a great deal in reality. This is why fate has the upper hand. On the other hand, Freud says, health allows the patient to be armed against the unhappiness about which they complain but which is common to everyone. Illness is the marker of the singularity of the patient at this border between fate and communal life. With the singularity of their illness given voice in psychoanalysis, perhaps one can give up the illness and join the rest of humanity. There is something important in this little vignette, which can sometimes sound too much like a process of adapting a patient's hysterical misery to the common reality of unhappiness as a means of settling down or—at best—a process of disenchantment. There is also something beyond the investment in being ill.

Lacan has said that an analysis changes nothing in reality yet changes everything for a patient. That is the difference between analysis and other therapies. What, he asks, is this everything that isn't reality? If we push this well-known fable further on the value of common unhappiness— one that seemed to alter little over the years, since it holds as much then as it does over thirty-five years later in *Civilization and Its Discontents* (1930)—Freud is not necessarily making the hysteric more reasonable or more of a common everyday human. At the point in *Studies in Hysteria* where he evokes this little parable, he is speaking about the confrontation with something impossible—with something at the limit—that surges up in treatment. He describes this as the obstacle that always arises in the course of treatment, namely, the transference to the analyst, the repetition of a spontaneous event that manifests in the relationship to the doctor.

The illness, the symptom, emerges here. This bodily event holds the key to the "everything" that changes in a psychoanalysis and brings a person back to life. If analysis is a question of knowing what exists, it must be done first on the inside, meaning inside the consulting room, then on the outside, one's singular pain in relation to a state of affairs in the wider world. Then and only then do we even know what universal malaise speaks through a symptom. We do not renounce illness but place it on the outside or into the analysis. Barring this confrontation, Freud says all he could have done was to have given the hysteric a new hysterical symptom.

While the symptom is originally accidental—accidentally caused in the course of history—its reappearance and intensification in psychoanalytic treatment brings it from the side of contingency to that of necessity. Psychoanalysis links contingency to necessity in the figure of urgency. This is Lacan's innocent or unknowing parent and the provoking presence of the analyst who will cause something to repeat, to manifest, and who will conjure this obstacle so that the patient "may know what exists" (1971–1972, 131) and what doesn't exist. For Lacan, this knowledge of one's symptom is perhaps the best description of the present that can possibly be given. This provocation of the analyst then has the function of spreading something critical in their symptom into their life as a whole, changing nothing in reality but everything for the patient. They will, according to Freud, feel "freer in the intervals" (Freud and Breuer [1895] 1995, 298), that is, between analytic sessions.

While the analyst may not be very free in this course of events, there is a pulsating, oscillating rhythm that analysis establishes, mirroring the symptom's game of *fort/da*—here, there, appearance, disappearance—that the patient can follow, ride along with, eventually siphoning a space of lesser misery, dropped preoccupation, creating "an order of the day which corresponds to the state of analysis" (298). "The symptom is on the agenda ... all the time," but it may find a way to breathe in a "to be continued" that seems to mark the space between sessions (298). A space of freedom from the symptom is established, or, rather, a freedom that was immanent to the symptom is made manifest. The symptom joins the conversation and seems to transform, extend even, into a space, a rhythmic way of being in the oscillations of thought, whose peaks dip "down into the unconscious—the reverse of what has been asserted of our normal psychical processes" (301). The norm is overturned. Conversion shows us how we may be converted.

Why this emphasis on conversion hysteria? Freud, many have noted, left hysteria behind, and most of his cases after Dora (1905) focus on men, obsession, phobia, and paranoia, only returning to the theme of femininity in 1931. Little is said about the body or conversion symptoms, save the controversial references to penis envy and castration anxiety. Penis envy comes up in the context of the problems analysts have ending a treatment, and while secondary gain is the context for a problem that the analysis itself created—one originally associated with conversion symptoms—at this late point, gain is rooted in the context of fantasy, clinging to infantile wishes as the final resistance of analysis, its so-called bedrock obstacle. Many will choose to remain ill rather than confront this bedrock loss, which is centered on acknowledging the help of the analyst. Time rears its head again. The symptom, if it fails to extend into its own unique time, grinds everything down in an impetuousness that makes the space of analysis unending. Freud's concept of universal malaise is here depicted as the half-converted state of an analysis caught in negative transference.

Nevertheless, conversion symptoms imply their own search for an end. Always on the agenda, always insisting and joining the conversation, Freud begins to transform his model of excitation and the quantitative or economic factors of the psychical apparatus on the basis of what he was learning from conversion hysterics. The symptom, he finds out, will not quit. And at the same time, it has entirely quit without delay. It leaves the psychical sphere, splitting the mind, and then makes a detour into the soma in order to insist there. The symptom leaves the psychic sphere separated off but intact. Conversion rearranges the psyche in order to wait, to allow the symptom to find an end, a solution.

When Freud compares conversion hysteria with anxiety hysteria (what we would think of now as everything that falls under the heading of anxiety disorders and panic) or even obsessional ideas, what becomes clear is that the split soma-psyche in conversion creates a pure symptom, if not *the* true symptom. The other symptomatic structures fail in their transformational relation to the psychical dimension, especially insofar as their defensive structure is simply too permanent. Psyche seems undefined, a kind of medial zone of incessant defense and substitution, projection and hallucination, what he eventually calls an unending series of half-measures. Freud almost depicts it as a kind of holding back of psyche from being properly psychical, a kind of anti- or antepsyche. In a letter to Fliess, while working on his unfinished "*neurotica*,"[1] Freud writes:

> If the symptoms of anxiety neurosis are examined more closely, one finds in the neurosis disjointed pieces of a major anxiety attack.... This is once again a kind of conversion in anxiety, just as occurs in hysteria ... but in hysteria it is psychic excitation that takes a wrong path exclusively into the somatic field, whereas here it is a physical tension, which cannot enter the psychic field and therefore remains on the physical path.
>
> (1985, 82)

Hysterical conversion is the reverse face of anxiety conversion, the former moving from the psychic to the somatic and the latter a failed movement from the somatic to the psychic. All the difficulty of working with what Freud labeled the actual neuroses follows from this failure of conversion hysteria.

A few letters later, Freud summarizes his findings in an elaborate chart. Hysteria appears as the only diagnosis with a satisfactory gain and with an unstable, rather than permanent, defense structure. The stable instability of the economics of conversion create a structure that acts like a sounding board responding to the note of a tuning fork, and this structure can become the space of the analysis. This is held out against the impotent screeching of anxiety, the sheer noise of paranoiac projection, and the hall of mirrors of obsession and compulsion. This is what we learn from Freud's first stab at a diagnostic system.

Freud's essay "The Neuro-psychoses of Defense" bears the strange subtitle "(an attempt at a psychological theory of acquired hysteria, of many phobia and obsessions and of certain hallucinatory psychoses)" ([1894] 1995, 45). The subtitle, both parenthetical and qualifying, seems to address the fact that the work was certainly not all he expected it to be. It was not comprehensive. This not-all quality, especially with so many strange and wonderful drafts that have come to light, is rather charming, while Freud's desire for a comprehensive theory is mostly distracting and comic. The 1894 paper is a sort of shrunken head in comparison to what Freud imagined of his *neurotica*, but it eventually transforms into the breathtaking project known as *The Interpretation of Dreams* (1900). Perhaps the one had to be dropped in order to become the other.

The associative and logical framework of the neuroses becomes the associative and logical framework of dreams. But we will never escape the stamp of Freud's early work mapping the neuroses. Not very much changes except his theory of anxiety. Hysteria, obsession, phobia (or anxiety hysteria), melancholia, and paranoia define the field. Hysteria assumes its place of prominence—both origin and end—despite its impending disappearance from Freud's investigative eye at the very moment when he reclassifies anxiety as prior to repression, not subsequent to it. Why? Perhaps it is enough for the moment to remember that one of the strange characteristics of hysteria is often a lack of anxiety, her *belle indifference*, which is not a far cry from the neutrality of the analyst. We need repression, the repression of anxiety and the creation of a symptom, whose hallmark transformation is signified by conversion. What is important here is the difference between repression—which is given a bad name by the dogmas that read the term politically—and suppression, which psychoanalytically speaking would be a better qualifier of what is making the most noise in every other neurotic structure aside from hysteria.

Agamben, picking up on the archaeological model in Freud through Ricoeur, notes the value of repression as the inability to replace an indestructible desire, an infantile scene, except by way of a repression that keeps it active. Repression becomes the "ordinary working condition" of psyche, a kind of delay where psyche always makes a late appearance (2009, 96). This allows for working over, even if that makes the mind vulnerable to the "infantile." Agamben here isn't seduced by any idea of the infantile as a regressive or primitive structure. Rather, this decisive latency in the subject creates belatedness, a temporal ordering that is workable, even the very condition of work. Agamben will use this Freudian temporality as a working model for his historical and genealogical study.

We must work with repression or, rather, see repression as a working condition—the only means through which one might reveal the present and not simply what clouds it. The rhythmic structure of hysteria is the preservation of a sounding board that remains in the body, gives body to psyche, and vice versa, value to material. It points to a world that otherwise remains latent or concealed but that erupts from time to time in symptoms attesting to something important in the here and now. The force of repression creates a new relationship to the way the hysteric relates to knowledge, namely, that she does not know, and this not-knowing—far from being a problem—becomes her virtue.

In the case of Dora, Freud compares listening to her history to trying to navigate an unnavigable river "whose stream is at one moment choked by masses of rock and at another divided and lost among shallows and sandbanks" ([1905a] 1995, 3). He wonders how anyone could produce a smooth and exact history with a neurosis whose main feature is a fragmentation of memory by virtue of repression. Neurotic narrative gaps, if not formed through the willing distortion of conscious shame, are formed by an uncontrollable unconscious resistance that arises in the act of speaking, wiping away intention, and/or by real amnestic holes into which past and present memories fall. The removal of symptoms and the restoration of memory form the bidirectional pathway of treatment: when one is reached, so is the other.

Hysterics are often judged for this functional fragmentation—"She remembers nothing! Certainly nothing accurately!" Remove the ideal of an unpunctured surface so that hysterical narrative can be seen instead to hold open certain possibilities. Freud, for one, extols the virtues of working with repression, not against it. And he certainly gave up trying to force a narrative from the get-go. Any fragment of a dream, no matter how small or incoherent, can work in the direction of analysis, and—as many analysts know—it can work even better than a dream remembered in total. Work, in the method of psychoanalysis, allows for forgetting. It is only consciously forgotten, after all.

When Freud returns to conversion hysteria again in his later work *Inhibitions, Symptoms, and Anxiety* (1926), he portrays the most intimate connection between what he calls repression, hysteria, and external anticathexis or "scotomization." What Freud means by this last term is the special kind of *not wanting to see* that the hysteric embodies, a paradoxical vigilance against certain perceptions. This hysterical configuration—characterized by her relation to amnesia or not knowing—moves in the opposite direction to obsessionality and phobia, which use regression and internal anticathexis. Theirs is a hypervigilance that keeps a blindness to one's unconscious life intact. Defense against the outside characterizes hysteria, while defense against the inside characterizes obsessionality and phobia.

Freud, at this late point, says that we must understand better how defense turned against the external world leaves the symptom and the personality of the hysteric intact, whereas the cost on the obsessional and phobic ego is much greater: "The reaction formation of hysteria clings tenaciously to a particular object and never spreads over into a general disposition of the ego, whereas what is characteristic of obsessional neurosis is precisely a spreading-over of this kind—a loosening of relations to the object and a facilitation of displacement in the choice of object" ([1926] 1995, 158). A woman, he says, will be tender to her children—whom she otherwise hates—but not necessarily tender to children in general or as a person. In the phobic or obsessional, it becomes characterological. They are creatures of reaction-formation rather than of symptomatic reactions to creaturely life.

The obsessional and phobic patients know what to avoid, and their ego identifies or adapts to the symptom. The old adage of the difficulty of treating ego-syntonic, or ego-friendly, symptoms, rears its head: how can you treat what doesn't cause distress? What is avoided is what is unpleasant, external, disavowed; they simply don't like it, they don't want it, they aren't it, it has nothing to do with them. Consolidation happens from the outside in. Add to this what Freud calls regression away from the libidinal and the erection of an internal fortress that undoes the force of libido (internal anticathexis), and we have, in a way, a pure defense against desire, against what is anarchic about desire.

For Freud, this structural difference is the difference of a fortification against the symptom from the inside as opposed to the structuring effect of the symptom itself:

> We have seen too, that in obsessional neurosis, anticathexis, which is also presumably present in hysteria, plays a specially large part in protecting the ego by effecting a reactive alteration in it. Our attention has, moreover, been drawn to a process of "isolation" . . . which finds direct symptomatic manifestation, and to a procedure, that may be called magical, of "undoing" what has been done—a procedure about whose defensive purpose there can be no doubt, but which has no longer any resemblance to the process of "repression."
>
> (164)

The obsessive and phobic patients distort their personalities or egos in order to buttress themselves against the symptom. The symptom is isolated in a stream of contradictory thoughts that have little to do with a reality that they are indifferent to and find undesirable at best.

The hysteric is the creation and preservation of the symptom. The conversion symptom, through repression and somatization, appears to be waiting for something. In particular, it appears to be waiting for something it wants to see in the external world. The symptom acts like a parasite on a host, unassimilable, foreign. Yet this symptom is opposed to all it does not wish to see. She scotomizes reality in order to keep her wishes alive. The hysteric is a lady in waiting. She doesn't know what she knows, what her symptom knows. She doesn't even know what it is that she is waiting to find. This constitutes the power of somatized amnesia.

One of the peculiar aspects of hysterical amnesias is that this way of being by forgetting allows one to begin again . . . and again. To try again to see or look for what their symptoms attest to. It is a constant twilight of the world, whose naïve power of charm is not lost on either those who experience it nor those who encounter it in another. She addresses the world around her. She sinks back from it. From what primordial darkness did the human creature emerge? What does she want? One need only watch the hysteric emerge and sink into an abyss to give shape to an answer. Freud certainly did. To forget is to inhabit another scene, an underworld, close to unconscious life. It is not only a life lived in daydreams but a vigilance that corresponds to wish.

Of course, always beginning again surely, at some point, defeats the idea of beginning—enter the psychoanalyst—but one must admit that on some level always beginning again has more potential than never beginning or always ending and bringing to a close. Closure, in the sense of locking consciousness in a framework set against the symptom, is the strategy of the obsessive and phobic structure. During Anna O's night fugues, she lived out the memory of the previous year in exact facsimile. She could begin again every night, calling in her precious Dr. B to witness this miracle of memory. The prior is priority. The past is seamless with the present. The symptom is able to remain on the agenda with all the affective urgency that belongs to it.

Analysis reconfigures a patient's priorities, perhaps close to the manner in which Freud wrote to Fliess about the attraction of others to saints (as opposed to what is naturally repugnant and unsociable about obsessions and phobia). He says that it is as if we were waiting for what has been stored up, what Freud called "the music of the future" (1985, 296). In a logic of love and identification, we identify with the saint's waiting, their waiting for the future, for their destiny. Of course, in this music, together with the hysteric's sounding board in her abdomen, we find simply another name for conversion disorder—Freud's hysterical unconscious. Linking these two moments, the early work on hysteria in the 1890s, to *Inhibitions, Symptoms, and Anxiety*, published in 1926, we find Freud presaging the current scotomization of hysteria and the preservation of conversion, quitting his investigation of the mysterious transformation of psyche into soma. This is Freud's music of the future.

THE ARCHITECTURE OF HYSTERIA

Let us take a closer look at Freud's early work on the architecture of hysteria. "In hysteria," he writes, "the incompatible idea is rendered innocuous by its sum of excitation being transformed into something somatic. For this I should like to propose the name of *conversion*" (Freud and Breuer [1895] 1995, 49). Through what Freud understands to be a false connection to the body that meets with somatic compliance, this innervation frees the ego from the contradiction of the incompatible idea. However, Freud carries on:

> It has burdened itself with a mnemic symbol which finds lodgment in consciousness, like a sort of parasite, either in the form of an irresolvable motor innervation or as a constantly recurring hallucinatory sensation, and which persists until a conversion in the opposite direction takes place. Consequently the memory trace of the repressed idea has, after all, not been dissolved; from then on, it forms the nucleus of a second psychical group.
>
> (49)

Hysteria is conversion hysteria because of this link to the somatic field and because of the complete conversion that takes place, decisively splitting the subject. It forms the nucleus of a second psychical system that acts like a sort of parasite, burdening consciousness. Conversion is extraterritorial.

This splitting of mind, however, is not the decisive feature; rather it is "the capacity for conversion." Freud says that conversion is "the psychophysical aptitude for transposing very large sums of excitation" (50). What we find is a process where there is a conversion in the direction of the body, a necessity for conversion as a demand coming from the ego, and a mnemic symbol that represents this transposition. All of this Freud calls an aptitude, an intimacy, nearly chemical. The insistent core of one's person that allows large sums of excitation to circulate continually and to construct an architecture—one that eventually comes to mirror the architecture of analysis itself.

What becomes fascinating is when one begins to consider the mnemic symbol not as demanding a conversion away from the body back toward the hallowed ground of the psyche but as a move from body to more body, as embodiment. The mnemic symbol contains the essence of body or is body in itself. It is soma to the second power, what later Lacanians will call the body-event that is conjured in analysis, namely, that which repeats through the transference (Miller 2015). If the ego is first and foremost a body ego, the projection of a surface, this projection is transformed into psychoanalysis itself, its own unfolding. Freud designated this possibility by the series of strange terms that indicate something folded on the inside—symptom, mnemic symbol, traumatic trace, pathogenic nucleus, and parasite. This radically other scene or territory can only be approached, step by step, fragment by fragment, and its connection to the body is not severed but rather harnessed. Everything in psychoanalysis that follows on the heels of affect evokes this terrain.

The successive layers of the ego, like those of an onion or the stratification of the unconscious, are similarly modeled in the psychic constellation of conversion hysteria. There is a layering of times in conversion, from the traumatic nucleus to other moments—what Freud called "auxiliary moments," which are inscribed around the nucleus. As this is reawakened, a series of links are established. Freud often wanted to label these events time one, time two, etc., setting up a series of chains. Two of the peculiar characteristics of hysteria were the necessity to proceed backward in time and the necessity that there be two times, that there be this connective link in order to awaken, *nachträglichkeit*, the slumbering pathogen.

This is a moment that seems to loop back on itself—from time one to time two, back to time one—with analysis proceeding in reverse direction, from time two to time one, back to time two. Past, present, past; present, past, present. "The distribution of excitation thus brought about in hysteria usually turns out to be an unstable one," though fortuitously so, since this potentially compels the subject to work over the idea associatively (Freud and Breuer [1895] 1995, 50). This is, of course, only the case when they do not entirely give in to hysterical attacks, to this massive discharge on the level of the body, reestablishing repression, bringing us back constantly to the disordering of time two sans time one.

What we see is that the intensifying rhythmic oscillations of analysis are borrowed from hysterical symptoms and partake in this prolonging of them in the direction of their working over. In fact, this may be a model for what Freud eventually calls *working through*, as distinct from remembering or repeating. But here, with the concept of conversion, I'd like to think of this working through as the formal affective turning of conversion rather than anything ideational, which tends to evoke the image of "finally" understanding. This takes a rather important concrete form in Freud's "Draft M—The Architecture of Hysteria" (1897; in Freud 1985, 246–48).

The model of analysis—from conscious recollection through associations, from the symptom to another surface, from the symptom to further stratification, from fantasy to the scenes that they mask, looping back around in order to move only further—is given an image. I, II, III, IV—these strata take their cue from the idea of an architecture of hysteria. Can we even imagine what analysis might look like if it followed the cadence of anxiety hysteria, paranoia, or the obsessional? The chronological and topological mapping that Freud depicts for us can be deceptive. Far from a seamless archeological dig, in "Draft M" he shows us the unconscious as composed of fragments, memories decomposed and then compounded like chemical bodies.

The body in bits and pieces is here the unconscious as a constellation of traces tied ever so closely with the sensory realm, what he would describe as intertwined "genealogical trees" or multiple nodal points in "The Aetiology of Hysteria." ([1896] 1995). It is for this reason that Freud felt that man's prehistory, which composed both the unconscious and

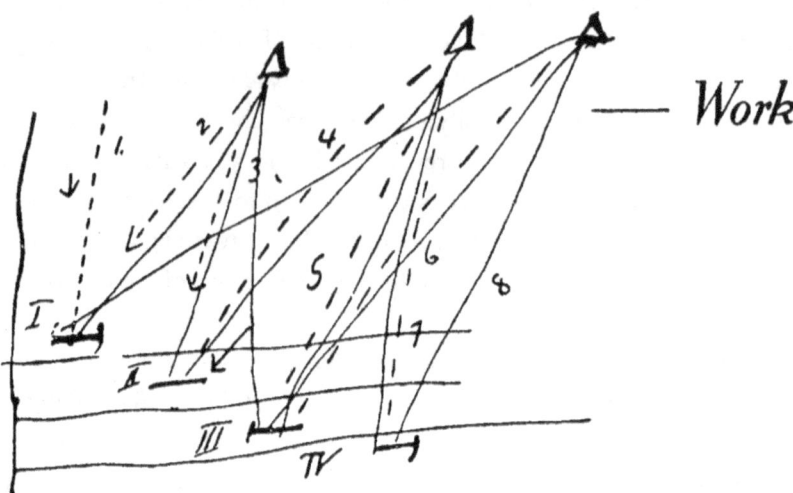

2.1 Untitled drawing from Freud's *Draft M: The Architecture of Hysteria*, included in his letter to Wilhelm Fliess, May 25, 1897.

Source: Reproduced by permission of The Marsh Agency Ltd. on behalf of Sigmund Freud Copyrights.

the amnesia analogous to hysterical amnesia, suggested to him that "what is seen in the prehistoric period produces dreams; what is heard in it produces fantasies; what is experienced sexually in it produces the psychoneuroses" (1985, 302). Thus, all chronological corrections, all scenes in total, are created by the action of consciousness. In the unconscious, we only have acoustic, visual, and mnemic fragments, whose offshoots—namely fantasies and symptoms—are formed by amalgamation.

The work of analysis is less an unearthing of trauma and more an act of deconstruction—the decomposition of symptoms and fantasies into their parts as the luminous fragments of an ancient body. Whether we add to this any chronology, meaningful or otherwise, is an act of construction or reconstruction; it is additive. But the work, as Freud pinpoints it here, is not the unearthing or reconstruction of ruins. The attempt at reconstruction is still a work of *Saxa loquutur!*, of making stones talk. This little-known region—open to translation, a series of stones, pieces of the life of the body—Freud would eventually call the field of the sexual accidents that form a life and the symptoms that are its means of continuation.

If we turn to what Freud says about the other psychoneuroses, the ones that lack the aptitude for conversion, what we find is that the affect or excitation is "obliged to remain in the psychical sphere" while the idea, "still left in consciousness," is separated from the process of association ([1896] 1995). Contrast this with conversion, where the affect is converted to the somatic sphere so that the idea can enter into repression, entering a system of unconscious association in a series of architecturally formed links. Of the obsessional structure, Freud writes that "its affect, which has become free, attaches itself to other ideas which are not in themselves incompatible; and thanks to this 'false connection,' those ideas turn into obsessional ideas. This, in a few words, is the psychological theory of obsessions and phobias" ([1894] 1995, 52). In other words, obsessions and phobias need the greater force of repression, one that requires a reopening onto the body rather than the easily found false connections of conscious association.

The transposition of affect, the flight of obsessional ideas, puts the obsessive or phobic patient at a disadvantage to the conversion hysteric. Everything remains in the psychical sphere, and "the relationship between psychical excitation and somatic innervation has undergone no change" (55). Conversion into the body creates a bodily system, an embodied unconscious mind, something not unlike "a series of electric charges spread over the surface of a body," without which it seems impossible to imagine either the clinical practice of psychoanalysis or our contemporary model of the sexual subject. From this is born the "limit" concept of the Freudian drive, meant to evoke this other territory (what he eventually calls the id), the dream and symptom as wish, and the transference as a repetition of the sexual accidents of life and their role in fantasy.

I cannot get away with talking about the body without talking about the *sexual* body in particular for much longer. The term "sexual" is entirely ambiguous, even when concrete. Certainly, in this early period of Freud's work the sexual is what is the most obscure while also the most literal. Freud's obsessions with *coitus interruptus*, abstinence, masturbation, and sexual abuse are well documented, especially in his letters to Fliess, to whom he serves up an equal dose of reports on sexual practices and all the small conversion disorders coursing through him and his family. Rather than move through the well-trod ground of trauma versus fantasy that seems to crown his early efforts of thought, a dichotomy that in any case feels like a drum that has been banged on with distracting vehemence over the last one hundred years, I will turn elsewhere, namely, toward melancholia.

There is a fascinating graphic representation that Freud conjures when comparing melancholia with hysteria in an earlier letter, "Draft G—Melancholia," to Fliess (Freud 1985, 100). Melancholia is a diagnosis that received scarcely any mention in his early papers, only reappearing much later in his much-celebrated "Mourning and Melancholia" (1917). Freud compares hysteria and melancholia on the grounds of a mutual history of (sexual) anesthesia, an inhibition at the level of the body that is important for Freud to grapple with. It may provide the key to inhibition—always sexual for Freud—which he is at pains to justify given his theory of the pleasure principle at the time he was writing. The graph is titled "schematic diagram of sexuality." We can see the somatic psychic field stretched between sensations and tensions in the organs and the boundary of the ego, whose extension into the external world only happens via the sexual object. Freud here gives representation to so much of what he was trying to map in this early period, and the idea that the sexual object, or the love object, is our only access to reality feels ever so literal in this diagram.

Lacan's circuit of desire, his topological model of the Klein bottle or the dissection of the torus into the figure 8, the Möbius strip, all bear a striking resemblance to this early graph of Freud's. Lacan's topological renderings were supposed to be taken as literal, the literal structure of the body—you are a tube, a sack, a knot! Working with these figures was meant to demonstrate the cutting effect of the analytic act, its structural reorganization of the patient, and the edge structure of the psyche. Freud's graph also indicates something of the place where he would like

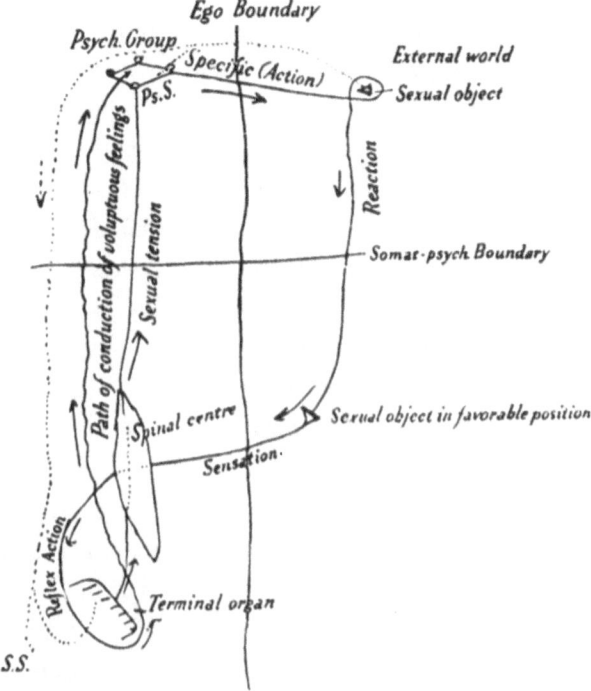

2.2 Drawing titled "Schematic Diagram of Sexuality" in Freud's *Draft G: Melancholia*, included in his letter to Wilhelm Fliess, January 7, 1895.

Source: Reproduced by permission of The Marsh Agency Ltd. on behalf of Sigmund Freud Copyrights.

psychoanalysis to intervene, and the model must be taken as literal, on the side of the body, and not an ideal.

In fact, we can almost see the body in the schema—genitalia, spine, head—stacked together to form a conduit for voluptuous feelings whose reflex arc wraps around its object. We pass through the soma-psyche boundary, attempting to break back into the body, where, as Freud writes, "the sexual object" is finally "in a favorable position" (1985, 100). This piece of the external world, created by an internal flow of sensations, is taken back inside. The object is then in a position to provide the psyche with feelings of pleasure—instead of mere tension and longing—through a reawakening in the somatic field. The finding of the object is always a sexual-schematic refinding. This idea of the circuit between a body and sexual object mirrors the trajectory of hysteria and the somatic break-in of the parasitic symptom.

We move from the somatic sexual, or s.S., to the psychic sexual, Ps. S., through V, voluptuous feeling or feelings of pleasure. Tension is converted to voluptuousness, a conversion that defines the mutability of the drive as it organizes the sexual field. Conversion here is both economic and psychical, form and content; it is the literal movements of the body that extend into the outside world. The image is like a conversion table, and Freud puts it to work in this draft, distinguishing his classical neuroses from the three different forms of melancholia that one witnesses in the clinic.

The most extreme melancholia is cyclic depression—what we now think of as bipolar disorder—and one can imagine the somatic system oscillating between a weakening and excess of libido. This is how the vegetative and manic symptoms are produced in an alternation between draining and flooding the psyche, between hallucinatory psychosis and total depletion. The fact that no one, not even the psychoanalyst, argues that depression is not on some level biological finds resonance here. It takes place in the body; it is a very real disordering. Without the tie to the love object in reality, the cord snaps, and the body folds in on itself. Nihilism and mania beckon as evidence of the rhythms of a closed loop, this unending interiority.

Neurasthenic melancholia—languor, malaise, boredom—Freud ties to excessive masturbation, namely, too much terminal discharge of sensation, creating an overall weakening of one's system. This is what we might think of as the vicissitudes of addiction and the problems of indulgence that eventually induce anesthesia. Here, depression follows an excess, but one that creates an inability to maintain any store of energy or pleasure that might amount to anything other than a demand for total discharge. Your system is spent. You've blown your load too many times—the result of a reified love object that you infinitely consume because it is not separate from yourself, tied into the external world.

Finally, Freud turns to somatic sexual sensations and tensions that are trapped at the border of psyche-soma, unable to transform in the psychical field, which is the very mode of anxiety in reality—you can't move freely across a boundary, you can't approach a certain threshold. When there is an additional loss of libido in the field of the psyche, we have the structure for anxiety melancholia. This is close to anxiety hysteria when it reaches the pitch of a mild melancholia, something that we see clinically all the time: anhedonia, alexithymia, and that strange admixture of anxiety and depression in response to the claims of love. One might call this simply the stronger vicissitudes of disappointment and disenchantment. Furthermore, Freud says that any neurosis that bears with it a low level of tension in the somato-sexual field takes on a melancholic stamp.

Freud here universalizes the mechanics of melancholia, which seems to cut through discrete categories. It is for this reason that melancholia is a difficult breed—its own clinical entity for sure—but one that finds its way into all the other structures when there is a quantifiable loss of libido that stamps one's system. A blow to the possibility for transformation, melancholia may even affect the overall aptitude or capacity for conversion. In fact, each configuration of melancholia speaks to a particular form of failure in relation to conversion symptoms.

It is fascinating that what is revealed beyond a phenomenology of pathology is the sheer economics of the libido. On this basis, Freud says that while anesthesia is possible without melancholia, melancholia is not possible without anesthesia. Anesthesia is defined by the omission of feelings of pleasure but is not necessarily found with the diminution of somatic sexual energy. Prolonged anesthesia, like accumulated deprivation—longing drawn out into its most painful pitch—paves the way for melancholia, defined by a diminution in pleasure, an impoverishment in psychic life, and the lowering of somatic excitation. The reaction to too much pain is often numbing; too much numbing creates the conditions for melancholia.

Freud likens the overall systemic loss in melancholia to a drawing in, an effect of suction that can reach the level of a massive psychic hemorrhaging, which can produce pain: "the uncoupling of associations is always painful" (1985, 103). The pain of melancholia and mourning is real, again a moment when soma and psyche are barely distinguishable. Freud wondered why something so inevitable would be so painful. It didn't intuitively make sense to him, since it overburdened both the psyche and the physical body. The best description of melancholia, writes Freud, is "psychic inhibition with instinctual impoverishment and pain concerning it" (1985, 102). Again, contrast this with the painless inhibition of the obsessional or the indifference of hysterical symptoms.

On the surface, there is an inhibition of mourning, a preoccupation with the longing for something lost, usually a lost object of love. Functionally, there is a loss of libido and an anesthetic history that has paved the way for the much graver condition of chronic melancholia. Freud says that we could perhaps think of melancholia as a longing for, and mourning of, a loss in one's instinctual life rather than any object in particular, emphasizing function over form. But how can we mourn a loss of libido? How can we mourn a loss as obscure as this, something enigmatic, formal, energic? Where does this work even begin?

Freud famously states that a loss in instinctual life defines the demands of civilization upon the individual. In this diagram, hysteria, anxiety, and melancholia are markers of the varying costs of civilized sexuality—where it squeezes the life of the body. These point to different levels of repression, stagnation, or anesthesia in relation to one's primary symptoms, which indicate the variety of paths of conversion. "Every man must find out for himself in what particular fashion he can be saved," writes Freud in *Civilization and Its Discontents* ([1930] 1995, 83–84) of the varied though specific solutions to the pleasure principle that each individual must create.

One can imagine that this is precisely why Freud eventually declares psychoanalysis to be antisocial, since it returns to the patient what civilization had attempted to exact from them:

> If the ethical restrictions demanded by society play a part in the deprivation imposed on the patient, treatment can, after all, give him the courage, or perhaps a direct injunction, to disregard those barriers and achieve satisfaction and recovery while forging the fulfillment of an

ideal that is exalted, but so often not adhered to, by society. The patient will thus become healthy by "living a full life" sexually. This, it is true, casts a shadow on analytic treatment for not serving general morality. What it has given to the individual it will have taken from the community.

([1917b] 1995, 432)

Much as psychoanalysis takes over the hysterical rhythms of the symptom, here the transformation of melancholia (in relation to a general malaise) takes the shadow cast on the ego—the loss that is preserved in the body—and instead makes it a stain on the profession as a whole. The patient is encouraged, if not given an injunction, to find the courage to push back against this price at all costs. So while hysteria is the model for the symptom, the through-line of melancholia in all psychoneuroses provides the model for the cure.

In hysteria, in contrast to melancholia, everything below the soma-psyche boundary is in working order, much as in conversion hysteria a secondary psychical system creates a preserved order. Hysteria is about linking, association, preservation, conversion, and excess stimulation—a hypersomatic field. Freud likened this marked territory to a nature preserve, and here, with this diagram of sexuality, what is preserved is the somatic field, which loses none of its vitality. The problem is simply that no one is enjoying it.

Voluptuous feelings are there but are not admitted to the psychical system or only arrive undercover, often in the form of disgust. This hysterical anesthesia is entirely analogous to hysterical anorexia, meaning disgust at the things we should otherwise take pleasure in, the things related to appetite. The hidden wish fulfillment (past or present) beckons—even if it is transformed into disgust—in contrast to melancholia, where the possibility of wishing isn't even present, having been lost in a tide of longing, deprivation, and diminution. The solution to melancholia, then, is not love but *more* hysteria. Why?

The answer is the body. In hysteria, there is a split—a radical one—that follows the lines of this soma-psyche boundary, which Freud called conversion disorder. There is a radical cut, unlike in melancholia, where the system takes a blow and everything remains trapped, stagnating. In hysteria the soma-sexual is intact—it is preserved. The conversion between psyche and soma holds psyche in reserve and preserves the force of the sexual. This is why the hysteric is so excitable, full of energy to the point of excess, and full of symptoms that respond to the day. Freud marvels at her for the virtue of this split because she is able to transpose somatic sexuality across the map—into psyche, into more body, into external love objects, into external hated objects, probably an infinite number of possibilities. Again, her peculiar "psycho-physical aptitude for conversion" (Freud and Breuer [1893] 1995, 50).

The hysterical symptom is a means of preservation and a place of pure potential. She is a lady in waiting, waiting with her claims to love, waiting for this object, which is something absolutely specific, exact, singular. This object is something that she will construct piece by piece. She searches for an answer; she surveys the surrounding world—waiting from the inside out, waiting for what she will allow or deign to allow to break in, rewriting soma from the outside in. And if she doesn't find the means to make it? There is, of course, the constant threat of melancholia.

If we push the logic of this schema, we might glimpse the ideal psychosexual arrangement, this beautiful vision of a preserved sexual order. As with all diagrams, this is nothing more than an ideal form, like most of Freud's iterations on the theme of adult genital sexuality. But Freud always posits this ideal in order to let it drop—this is his method—and we should read in his schema a certain kind of promise. A promise in line with the conversion hysteric, a promise that this structure of conversion is the possibility that the world will be rewritten, will turn inside out, will be converted by her. This emptied promise is the hysterical promise of psychoanalysis.

Following this table of conversions, psychoanalysis seems modeled on hysterical conversion as the potential conversion that comes on the heels of pleasure, opening the narrow straits between whatever is constituted as psyche and a preserved body. Desire—full throttle—with all its urgency retained must be admitted into the psychic realm. Desire remains tied to the body, carrying the drives forward. Melancholia and the malaise of civilized life and morality stand at the other pole to hysteria, and through the psychoanalytic cure, we take the hole in one's psycho-somatic life—whatever loss is contained therein—and stage an encounter with it in the external world. We have to force both desire and this hole onto the outside. She has to do this without the action resulting in either psychosis or hysterical hallucinatory confusion.

The ill-defined term "sublimation" hovers here in the background, a concept Lacan says Freud's mouth remained sewn shut about. The one qualification of sublimation that Freud ventured was that while sublimation leaves repression intact, it manages to bypass it economically, bringing with it a full experience of satisfaction. The gap between one's aptitude and one's ideal is the space in which the neurotic person usually founders. This gap closes momentarily in sublimation at the point of experienced pleasure, in the externalization of a desire that is forced into the world.

Mystical experiences, apophantic judgments like oracles, epiphanies, and the work that comes from the regression of a psychoanalytic treatment, meet with psychosis and hysterical confusion or delirium at the hinge of the felt polarity bearable-unbearable. Psychotic breakdown and sublimation are both results of a disordering on the level of the body, of this movement of huge quantities of energy or drive-life. But only one has the force of conversion because in being able to bear it, it can be borne. Freud's own conversion disorder (as well as his depressive lethargy with respect to his life as a doctor, husband, and father) cleared after writing *The Interpretation of Dreams* (1900), which he called his seedling, a *nova species mihi*, new species of me—Freud's autoconversion, his self-conversion of a *petite* conversion hysteria and mild melancholia.

III

FATHER CAN'T YOU SEE

Thus so many images speak to us, "sleep in a nest of flames . . . really drunken sleep on the shore . . . sea mixed with sun," as well as "I was idle, prey to a heavy fever" . . . the need to say everything in the time of a bolt of lightning, foreign to the faculty of saying that needs duration. Enough seen. Enough had. Enough known.

—MAURICE BLANCHOT, *THE WORK OF FIRE*

FATHER CAN'T YOU SEE

In a state of belligerent unhappiness, I began reading horoscopes late into the night, as if they were lullabies. Only exhaustion and the force of sleep could make me stop. These horoscopes are often in broken English—they are the music of the future, written by machines overseas. These messages don't say anything. They are prophecies of nothing. At best, they survey the landscape simply by speaking to you. Whispers and caresses, warnings and injunctions, a response to a longing that isn't even quite a longing to know or predict anything. This is the comfort. This is the exchange. Please over-see me.

It is miraculous to find speech so empty, proliferating in a virtual ether, sent to you, a point of origin formalized as a constellated expanse of sky that forever shifts, able to be marked by a date, your birth! What I find even stranger still is that these oracles do not function as a call—not to arms, or action, or anything in particular. It is not the call of religious conversion. It mimics the religious call but empties itself out. What I seem to ask for in reading these overdetermined stars is fundamentally intransitive in its request. What I receive is anonymous and provides no content. It is a purely formal exchange. What does it mean to look to be addressed? What porosity do the stars promise when taken as a predictable system of signs or, inversely, the emptying of a sign so that it is bereft of any signification whatsoever? That we may all together turn?

Individual and universe are found together, founded on nothing—or at least nothing real—insofar as it is simply a moment of contact. A question about how to read this communication hinges, again, on a question of knowledge. Here we find two faces of conversion: one I might call psychoanalytic, an ambiguous force of turning and calling; the other, something more religious, fundamental, a form of radicalization that must be foreign to psychoanalysis, which still, after all these years, is not a weltanschauung. We have a horoscope as a promise of nothing—but a promise nonetheless—and a horoscope as a certain promise, dictating a future and decisive actions.

I had a dream the other night. In it, he said to me, "I'm going to read you a letter where I ask to leave you." Or was it, "I ask you to leave?" I can't remember. There was some doubt or hesitation in the dream text at this point. What's the difference between the two statements? The direction taken by the object? The nature of the request as it reflects on the speaker's intentions? There is a question of motion. For the object: still there but almost alone, soon alone, or soon leaving, sent away, cast-off. She is left, or she is asked to leave. She is standing in the same place though the conditions have changed, or she must go elsewhere. Either way, the action is one of separation.

On the other hand, the subject's position seems to remain exactly the same. The I is firm: I am going to read to you. I am going to ask you. He is the one writing the letter. She is the one written upon, impressed. Asking someone to leave is different from asking *to* leave. The latter implies a moment of hesitation in the leaving other. Why ask? What permission is needed? Perhaps that was precisely the wish followed by the sense of ambiguity or question. Better that it be the former, the original dream thought, the request or appeal to leave. And somehow upon waking I introduced a doubt concerning the dream text, which was transformed through an act of rephrasing in the vein of greater certainty and violence. *I ask you to leave* arrives just as I leave the dream. It is a way of closing the dream off through conscious doubt, through an impending absolute.

My response—inside or out of the dream, it isn't clear—were these words: "Show me the dates. Show me what is mine and yours." The date-line, like a meridian on a globe, divides the field. Somehow the date is the final force of separation. I speed up the action. Here I am, there you are. This is what came before and this after. The date marks. Show me. I ask to make obvious what is hidden in the letter, the essence of the letter itself, its point of suspension. So while there is the wish—not to be left or asked to leave, or to leave or be left—and the precipitation of knowledge or understanding, this is not the only conclusion or line of interpretation.

The dream also creates movement, a choreography stretching from hesitation to a defined action where the final term moves from passive to active, from the future progressive to the future perfect. Separation is incarnated as movement. I also do not fail to hear the reference to sexual difference, to the child's game of "I'll show you mine if you show me yours." Whenever doubt appears in a dream, Freud says we must look for the perception of sexual difference. This sexual division "mine and yours" is also a division of the playing field. There is the position of author, the one who reads or writes, and there is the addressee, the one who is read to or written upon. The dream transforms subject positions into potentially occupied places—this is mine, and that is yours. Static at this extreme point, it hints at an unbearable sadness present in all sexual relationships.

The movement in the dream can be found not only in the play of subject-object positions but also in the linguistic form of call and response. It feels like a dialogue of translation or transcription. I'm going to read you this letter. Show me the dates. I'm going to ask to leave you. What is mine and what is yours. Perhaps then we might combine these, making the wish the original one—the one touching earliest childhood, the efflorescence of sexual curiosity and a first means of research—reaching out to the other. Show me. Even if the body is there as something engendered in the dream, a memory of bodies in their epistemophilic excitement, the dream is a series of word-feelings, more so even than a series of images. These words can be given or lost, received or rejected. What's mine is yours, and what's yours is yours. What's yours is mine, and what's mine is mine.

Rather than the territory being something established in advance, the exchange begins to mark the territory as it explores the field, pushing toward an unknown limit. It is looking for a date. In Latin, "date" is derived from *dare* and *data*, meaning to give, to deliver. Only in the nineteenth century does the word come to mean a romantic liaison, playing on its more general use to denote an appointment. I am interested in the sense of destiny or fate that is longed for, the meeting of all meetings, the force of deliverance, reached for in this dream through the other, through letters. To place this desire for deliverance at the heart of an erotic understanding of epistemology returns to something critical to the field of knowledge: the religious sense of conversion hiding inside a psychoanalytic or chemical variant.

The dream analysis points to a formal engine in the dream—anticipating a moment of deliverance in the Foucauldian sense, where in reaching forward it also reaches back, beyond the infantile, toward the first movements of freedom, until it coincides with the trajectory of existence itself. The useless, impossible self-reference of the "I" in "I am writing you a letter" is displaced into a reading, leaving, dating, showing, marking. The dream traverses a series of crucial figures: passive, active, away, here, left, lost . . . until it reaches the point where a date is asked for, an encounter, now. This is one way of defining destiny.

Too much separation makes circulation impossible. Too much closeness, and there is nothing to give. Both ends of the spectrum start to eclipse any bodily presentation, any immediate presence. The dream is a dream of will in and of itself: read, ask, leave, show, mark. The dream is thus not only the fulfillment of a wish; it is the formal presentation of fulfillment moving beyond all phantasmatic traces of the past that try to bring wishing to a halt. Agamben characterizes the dream this way: "This dimension beyond images and phantasms toward which the movement of the imagination is directed is not the obsessive repetition of a trauma or of a primal scene, but the initial moment of existence when 'the originary constitution of the world is accomplished'" (2009, 105).

There is another, earlier dream—words only also—that I heard or awoke with. Again, said to me, *I would if I could.* How unnecessary it is even to have to add that he couldn't. Can't. It doesn't need to be said. And it isn't clear if saying it is crueler than not. Here one seems to choose between a negation or a truncation, a statement of intention left in ellipse, rather than the force of an explanation, a justification, and a closing down. The dream's *yes,* its wish, is barely there but marked "I would," which is shadowed by the most painful of negations, if . . . not. There isn't even qualification. *Wouldn't* and *can't* define the space of the negative from the withholding of possibility to impossibility itself. All the vicissitudes of conflict and deficit that haunt psychiatry and psychoanalysis rear their head behind this dream.

In the end, we are left with a question of what is impossible or possible or what it is that defines these spaces: would not and cannot. The wish is followed by a wound, a dance between hysteria and melancholia, weaving the text at hand. We often break at the ambiguity of this dividing line. It isn't clear what is real, meaning impossible. It isn't possible to know what to reconcile if we don't know what to reconcile ourselves to. What reality? Whose reality? Why does this other confuse the field with the "I would," if they cannot? What can and can't be done? This has to be constructed by the one who receives the message.

The rules, by which I mean structure, and wish, by which I mean desire, are established through the interpretation of the dream. They do not exist a priori. In fact, I think that "won't" and "can't" are the same. The dream is trying to collapse them so that they form a limit instead of a judgment, a wound, or a presupposition. It shows the subject as the one presented with something irreparable. If you won't, there is no difference from can't, and if you can't, there is nothing to be done. It is what it is.

Here the absolute *no* that haunts the dream could meet with a *yes*—a yes to this impossibility that arrives concealed, and whatever possibility there is, it is not something that can be determined in advance. But far from blind hope, it requires the confrontation with a limit. For Agamben, this is precisely what requires the most work, "seeing something simply in its being-thus-irreparable, but not for that reason necessary; thus, but not for that reason contingent—is love" (1993, 102.4). Love, then, is the separation that comes from touching the impossible—if you won't, you can't. If I wish otherwise, I must leave. We either set a date, or we don't.

If there is any reason why Freud's "*neurotica*" was transformed into *The Interpretation of Dreams* (1900), perhaps it is because he had to establish the wishing subject—the one encountered in the dream text—before he could outline the rules of the game. In any case, isn't it true that all of Freud's rules had to be overturned and that in the end, the rules of psychotherapy were the ones made by his conversion hysterics: "say what comes to mind?" Aren't they the ones to show this ever-evolving playing field?

If we take this one step further, what *The Interpretation of Dreams* does is not to explain dreams per se but to provide us with a model of psychoanalytic conversion, because it will always be the text that is both the origin—as both birth and act—of psychoanalysis at the same time that it is a text on dreams. It is an event that establishes a line, a limit, a date, where what came before and what follows will be marked. It is for this reason that I so closely link this original act of founding the field of psychoanalysis to an idea of conversion—a dazzling moment of disclosure that unites an original trace with a moment of anticipated freedom.

Lacan (1991) read Freud's report of the "Father, can't you see that I'm burning?" dream in exactly this way. But he left out that it was a hysteric's dream, transcribed, redreamt, heard in a lecture on dreams from her professor, its original source remaining to Freud unknown. The dreamer of this dream, the dream's originator, comes to inaugurate chapter 7 of *The Interpretation of Dreams*—certainly the cornerstone chapter for psychoanalysis—as a mystery. Presumably, some father who has lost a child, a fact that potentially means he is no longer a father. The dream is some dream by a man, repeated by another man, a professor . . . that becomes a dream by a woman told to Freud, her doctor. Oddly enough, it seems to recreate the scene of Freud's specimen dream—Irma's injection—that opens the dream book, a dream where a series of men attend to a wound in Irma's mouth wherein Freud disappears.

The dream reported by Freud's female patient hardly seems to be anything but a direct repetition of the original dream. The dream is from the perspective of the father, and Freud treats it as the dream of a father. The woman—her place in the dream, her rewriting of the dream—is seemingly absent. Freud states that the woman who redreamt it took only some elements of this dream in order to express her agreement on one point. But he never says what point that is or which elements she used. With what did she want to express her agreement? And what do we make of Freud's fascination with this dream that eclipses her own? Show me what is mine and yours . . .

For Freud, the point of the dream was to show how reality entered into the dream—the fire, the body of the burning child whose watchman had fallen asleep on him while his father slept—to allow this father to keep sleeping, to not see the reality in front of him in order to see his child one last time. To wake up is "to shorten his child's life by that moment of time" (Freud [1900] 1995, 510). This seems to encapsulate more of Freud's point than perhaps the hysteric who redreamed the dream, a point Freud wants to make about the place of perception in the psychological process of dreaming. Reality combines with wish—which is a retranslated reality, a converted reality—that Freud will call psychical reality. It is this that Lacan emphasizes in his interpretation of the dream, the point in the dream that he calls the Real, but a different real than Freud's perceptual reality, far from the reality that is happening outside. Fire outside versus fire inside.

Lacan's Real is not only something indicated by psyche but a point of the utmost cruelty, marked in this dream by the incomprehensible grief over the death of one's child. Wish and loss condense in the words of approbation said from child to parent, "Father, can't you see that I'm burning?" to this father who is asleep. Hear-again. Bits of visual and acoustic memory become fragments of persecution; the child is encountered one last time, loss undone, only to chastise one last time this father for having failed, for having let him die. This is the reality that the father wakes up to or, rather, the reality that the father wakes up from.

Lacan says this dream does not seem to prove that the dream is a wish—unless it is the wish to keep sleeping, in which case we have to ask: What wakes the dreamer up? Is it not another reality altogether—one's inner psychic reality, this burning body—that the dreamer wishes to escape? If this dream can get so close to the reality that causes it, the words coming from this dead child, Lacan asks: Is it not this reality *in* the dream, rather than the reality outside of it, that wakes us? Every dream at bottom is a nightmare. A trial by fire. Is there not more reality in this sentence, "Father, can't you see that I'm burning?" Lacan says, than in the fire in the next room whose light penetrates sleeping eyes? Is this not the point—the place where these words cover over an abyss—that the hysteric takes over? Is it here where she literalizes her symptom?

There is no father. He is a mystery. This child's words will echo in the psychoanalytic chamber for eternity, repeated by a woman, and then by Freud, one more time. "This sentence is itself a firebrand—of itself it brings fire where it falls and one cannot see what is burning for the flames blind us to the fact that the fire bears . . . on the real" (Lacan 1981, 59). It is too much. Freud will move on to the forgetting of dreams. In reality, Lacan says, there is only the missed encounter. The father is asleep. They are all asleep. A candle has fallen. A child is being burned. The dreamer is missing. The dream is someone else's dream.

This is so, yet in the dream there is a unique encounter—this reality that must be produced by the dream through "repeating itself, endlessly, in some never attained awakening" (59). The proliferation of fire: We are forced to do it again and again, to dream again and again, to try to coincide with another reality behind or beyond the dream itself. Is this the reason for the hiatus of the symptom—its ever-renewed wish? Is this the wish for something missing in order to continue to desire, or the very evocation of lack itself—a hole—with only a thin patina of words for shelter? It is both wish and wound—or better, the dream attempts to force their reconciliation.

Once the sentence has been uttered—I am burning—Lacan says that there is something here formally close in character to Freud's analysis of the Irma dream as a condensed formula of desire, what he named the writing on the wall. This formula, one that literally says that the dream is a wish, establishes the transference to Freud as the originator of psychoanalysis that will carry the field forward. These are the words of Freud at the edge of a hole, at this moment of rebirth. Far from these being simply indictments of the impossible situation of psychoanalysis forever tied to this man, they outline a possible freedom: I am burning, I am this wound, I am this voice from beyond. The wish for circulation, like that across the fields of Freud's diagram of sexuality, is a wish for movement sans inhibition, across boundaries, contained in these phrases composed of fire. But we cannot forget that at bottom, the formula for desire in Freud's Irma dream is also a stand in for semen—for a bodily product—and the burning child is nothing other than a statement about his having died from fever, the imagined torment of a body before death.

In Lacan's interview of a psychotic patient at the Hospital Sainte-Anne, a case named "A Lacanian Psychosis," Lacan (1980) speaks with a patient he calls a "rare bird," translating his name.[1] The patient, when explaining himself to Lacan, talks his way into a strange conundrum of not knowing if he feels without boundaries or whether he exists in the machinations of a solitary circle. In which configuration are you freer? While the patient seems more and more confounded, Lacan is quick and doesn't spare him: there is nothing to worry about. You live in a closed space. More freedom would actually do you well.

The rare bird isn't so sure. He complains of telepathy. Of the burden of having to know what everyone is thinking. He knows what the members of the audience are up to. Tell me, Lacan implores with some cruelty. He says he doesn't like the makeup of a woman in the audience, which, in a flash of lightning, Lacan transposes back to the patient. Have you worn makeup? Yes, he says. He was hoping to experience what it felt like to be a woman. The gap between hoping and experiencing feels encouraging to Lacan. You are hoping to get out, then! So it would seem that the answer to the conundrum is that the boundary is actually all too strong. There is no difference between a dream at night, Lacan says to the patient, and a waking dream. They are all your own ideas. We are all looking for the way out.

The patient suddenly recounts his first experience of hallucination: "I was masturbating, and I felt an extreme enjoyment. I had the sensation of rising into the air. Did I really rise, or is it an illusion of orgasm? From the point of view of thought, I really think that I levitated" (38). It isn't clear whether the rare bird's question is a question at all. The sensation of rising up, levitating, potentially closes the circle for good. His experience of erection is transformed into the idea of levitation. The certainty of the sensation of levitation becomes equivalent with the point of view of thought—from above as it were—and is in danger of becoming a certainty. Yes, I did levitate. Lacan seems to suggest that there must be another point of view than this one, one that presumably resides somewhere closer to this rare bird's questions about the illusion of orgasm and the wish to be the woman that he isn't. He is speaking to the difficulty of experiencing extreme enjoyment, something that even the neurotic has trouble questioning.

This doubling between orgasmic enjoyment and the sensation of rising up from the point of view of thought frustrates Lacan. "Yes, one does hope," he retorts, and then, seemingly hopeless himself, asks the patient what his plans are for the future (39). The rare bird sends Lacan's hope back to him: "I have hope of finding my power of judgment again" (40). The rare bird almost seems to anticipate Lacan's disappointed desire in this little conversation. Lacan wishes him luck. The rare bird leaves the room. But didn't this psychotic patient heroically ask about his own experience? He seems to say that he knows the difference between thought and judgment, even if the latter has escaped him for a time. That he would like to find a way.

Lacan, in a final gesture, turns to the audience and condemns this poor man. He says to them that it's only "getting worse for him." The telepathy has him in despair. "I don't see how he is going to get out of it. There are suicide attempts that end up succeeding. Yes" (41). It isn't clear if the *yes* is said with the intonation of a question or an exclamation. Either way, the words are damning. Even if hope circulates between these two, Lacan and a Lacanian psychosis, the only success—the only act that succeeds—is suicide. Yes.

One does hope. Some do commit suicide. Lacan, in *Television* ([1973] 1990), said we must translate the question "what may I hope for?" to "from where do you hope?" From the inside with a view to the outside? From the outside looking for how one might reenter? This hope is a hope for circulation, part of the hysterico-melancholic pathos, concretized as a belief in telepathy. The inside and outside are neither distinct realms but something, as Lacan wanted to demonstrate, painfully knotted, poised on a rim. The question of getting out, indeed of suicide, is the wrong way to ask the question. We are all hoping to get out, even the psychotic.

From my perspective, this patient on display speaks with a gentle clarity about his predicament—there are some things that we feel as if we can really believe from the point of view of thought. And when we begin to believe in this way, there is a question about whether one needs a firmer boundary or whether the trouble resides in being so completely locked in. Some judgment is necessary here. But of what nature? The feeling is deceptive. He knows this, yet he still, as he says, loses himself—"I can't manage to get hold of myself" (Lacan 1980, 40). For Lacan, the problem is always about separation, about structure. Judgment requires it. Thought is something else. Thought is always a trap.

Anything can be believed, especially from the trap that is the point of view of thought. Psychoanalysis has to work differently. The rare bird's telepathy, this collapsing of distance or failure of separation, is damning. It makes him want to commit suicide, and the only thought that pulls him back, so he says, is the idea that there is more to know, which arrives as a sentence that saved him as a teenager: "Life as a means of knowing" (37). Wanting to know is indeed Lacan's version of psychosis, since it never saved a soul, aside, perhaps, from our rare bird. Or maybe it didn't save him? Maybe it made him a Lacanian?

I had a dream the other night of a woman singing, full volume, "I'll never see you again" behind a screen, an inverse song to that of the presence of the burning child. I am a little closer to the reality of loss, unburdened by the added sting of conscience spoken to the father by the dead child, like salt in a wound. I was and wasn't asking for one more time. The song was simply the truth of what it means never to see something again, to have to sing it, both parties half obscured, reduced to song, on the edge of madness. There is a boundary in place so that there can be a place for wish—for the transcendence of song—which is in fact not transcendence at all except in its freedom to wish, which is why the dream just barely escapes being a nightmare.

This dream image followed on the heels of a dream image of women walking, head down, across the wing of plane. An ancient funeral procession, they walked without looking toward the edge, the sun a blinding brilliance at their backs that I felt as a sensation of warmth on my face. I said to the pilot, "I want what we were," which in saying it marked the object as impossible, already gone, dated. Mine and yours were a "we" for a moment, once upon a time. The wish was a purified wish in its stated impossibility. I knew that the wish was impossible. It was simply a question of saying it, knowing desire is felt the most strongly when it faces what was. The separation has already happened, even if the attachment, the desire even, remains.

What is comical is that in the middle of the night, bleary eyed, I frantically Googled "out on a wing" and couldn't understand why there wasn't anything but some bad 1970s country song on YouTube. Isn't it a common colloquial phrase? Only when I woke up the next morning did I realize that what I was looking for was "out on a limb." This metonymic shifting between limb and wing, from tree to bird, already prefigures the movement of the procession, the need implicit in mourning, the lengths to which one must go—somewhere between being out on a limb and winging it. Closure beckons, and wing walking or keeping something in the wings—one's wingman, as it were—is the refusal to give up the object. Between these two, the time signature of the object is being mapped in this space, which unfolds as the subject progressively disappears. Not suicide but syncope and song. Not levitation but a funeral procession. The utterance *I'll never see you again* may be better read as a statement about the object that one is when one relinquishes, finally, the attachment to the other.

One last dream. I am looking at a man who has died. The room is full of mourners. I ask an older gentleman a question about him and he says to me, "We will not say anything else. When someone dies, we close them, and cast them into the river of peace." I looked to see if they were going to close his eyes, which I realized was a rather childish interpretation of what was said, a silly literalizing, but nonetheless, there is a logic in children's misapprehensions. It felt as if what was said would have to be something that takes place on the body, not embodied speech as such but speech literalized, read to the letter.

Perhaps there is an identification with Freud's dream of his father's death and the ambiguous and ambivalent command—you are asked to close *the eyes*, which may also be *an eye*. Closure must have a material component, the link between looking for it and ceasing to look; closing the eyes was some part of a truth about the fact that closing takes place in the body, much as opening does—this strangely felt rhythm of the unconscious. Closing the eyes, the least material or tactile of the senses, opens the way to a feeling in the body that is linked with the movements of mourning. Separation, sensing that there as a limit, is felt as an endpoint.

I have also been called, by the likes of fathers, a disturber of the peace. If this indictment of being a disturber of the peace has made me angry in the past—something I've turned around on the other as a statement not about myself but as something concerning their own desire to be free of desire, which will never leave anyone in peace—in this dream, at least, I take it in. Peace is not simply the escape from desire but something about what it means to close one's eyes, about bringing something to an end, about the outer limit of any wish. The will to counterattack quiets.

I woke up from the dream thinking about the hell of revision, revisionist history, the endlessness of interpretation, the obsessive attempt to go over one's life or another's, this problem in psychoanalysis. When it is not a problem, it is more like something that erupts in the body and brings thinking to a close. Let the dead be dead. We will not speak any more about it. I'll never see you again.

In any of these dreams or psychoanalytic stories the question of the body is not one where it is something simply there, a body from which thinking takes flight, but rather as something that is evoked, provoked, and erupts, disrupting thought and opening onto another terrain. This point, nodal as Freud tended to call these affectively charged moments, seems to organize and formally structure the dream itself. It is important to me that we see this constellation together—body, affect, signifier—as the wishing subject that emerges from the dream, in the same way that it inaugurated the field of inquiry called psychoanalysis with the 1900 publication of Freud's *The Interpretation of Dreams*.

Reading, leaving, burning, levitating, walking, being blinded, or casting, or closing, all reveal the body of the wishing subject in a state of desire, reaching out toward the other from whom they are irrevocably separated. The body appears in this way with a hint of mourning—that is, when it is not saturated with it. Separation is not a fact or a state of being but something that must be made manifest not just once but again and again and again, in a work that I call psychoanalysis, conversion. This is the empty promise we psychoanalysts have to offer—your forever horoscope, your birthright and destiny.

IV

NEVER THE RIGHT MAN

(In Vancouver as the dark winter tapered into spring
I undertook to sing
My life my body these words
The men from a perspective.
For all those who confuse
Flirtation with monogamy
I drain the golden glass
They exist and glance upwards
Adjust their little caps)

—LISA ROBERTSON, POSTSCRIPT OF
THE MEN: A LYRIC BOOK

NEVER THE RIGHT MAN

Freud's "The Taboo on Virginity" ([1918] 1995) is perhaps one of his strangest papers, one where the conundrums of femininity and sexuality meet in a tale about virgin women and love. The paper helps us explore the concept of conversion, which sits at the heart of Freud's question about the change that must take place from the state of virginity to becoming a sexual being. Characteristically, Freud considers the question first through its failures: from societal biases, male fantasies, general inhibitions and fears, and what he defines as a particular resistance on the part of "some" women.

In the reverse direction, the concept of conversion helps us read this paper and the tangled thoughts of Freud whenever he broaches the dark continent, giving us a sense of what he is after beyond his own misogynistic misapprehensions and fixations on this bodily event, the supposed loss of virginity. The general landscape of sexual inhibition and resistance, sexualities restricted or left latent, speaks more broadly to the problem of dissatisfaction and to in-vogue diagnoses from anorexia to alexithymia, sexual anxieties—manifest in painful intercourse, frigidity, impotence, and other symptoms—and asexuality. I will tie this paper to Freud's thoughts on love and mass psychology and to the resistance to psychoanalysis, and to women, by civilization as a whole.

"The Taboo on Virginity" is part of Freud's trilogy on the psychology of love. Freud seems unable to write the female counterpart to "A Special Type of Choice of Object Made by Men" ([1910] 1995) and "The Universal Tendency Towards Debasement in the Sphere of Love" ([1912] 1995), writing *Totem and Taboo* ([1913b] 1995), "On Narcissism" ([1914] 1995), and "Mourning and Melancholia" ([1917a] 1995), among many other works, before he could finish the series with "The Taboo on Virginity" eight years later. The "Taboo" essay feels completely aberrant from the other two on men, which are both beautifully constructed and by now well-known essays interrogating the debasement of women and the tendency in men toward a Madonna-whore complex. The female counterpart essay on virginity meanders and is full of wild leaps, odd indictments, and, one must admit, bizarre conclusions. It has largely been ignored likely because it conjures the specter of Freud's misogyny—too offensive in that way that people find Freud offensive when it comes to women.

In fact, Freud does seem to be running into trouble in this essay, as he always does when he writes about women after the Dora case. It is almost as if he needed to write about narcissism and melancholia in order finally to write about women and love. This is a construction, of course, a gesture, but it is one I would like to make, rescuing this paper from the dustbin. In our earlier investigation of conversion, looking at "Draft G—Melancholia" in Freud's letters to Fliess (Freud 1985, 98–105), we saw how he links melancholia with hysteria through frigidity or sexual anesthesia, and this is what plagues Freud in the "Taboo" essay as well. "Draft G," "Mourning and Melancholia," *Totem and Taboo, Group Psychology and the Analysis of the Ego* ([1921] 1995), and "The Taboo on Virginity" can be read together as taking on a question of sexual anesthesia or, more broadly, inhibition and conversion. These papers link the failure of conversion in the form of inhibition and resistance to the failure of the sexual relationship.

Freud situates inhibition in relation to the properties of anesthesia, what he calls a loss of libido. You can be anesthetic—that is, suffer a loss of libido—without being melancholic, but you cannot be melancholic without being anesthetic or without a prolonged and excessive relation to this melancholic loss in libidinal life. This loss in libido is a consequence of resistances or inhibitions that have not been overcome. There is work left undone.

Freud says that much like hysteria, melancholia requires not necessarily the mourning of a particular object, of love, in this case, but what he calls mourning a loss of libido. The loss of libido first appears as symptomatic hysteria. This ongoing mourning is also a task for the virgin. Here Freud turns away from the love object to the question of libido, something that might be of particular relevance today with the resurgence of hysterical symptoms that come from the attempts to control libido—anorexia, anhedonia, and asexuality, to name a few. But how can one mourn a loss of libido? Very Freud. Very strange. Let's turn to the "Taboo" paper.

Freud begins with the idea that the demand for virginity in marriage is the demand that the girl will bring with her no memory of sexual relations with another. He calls this the "logical continuation of the right to exclusive possession of a woman, which forms the essence of monogamy, and the extension of this monopoly to cover the past" ([1918] 1995, 193). As a diagnosis of monogamy, it is absolutely brilliant. Freud continues, saying that from this perspective we can understand what had originally looked like a prejudice in our views on women's erotic lives. The man who is able to overcome all her resistances, all her impulses so long held in check, to satisfy her desire for love, will be the man that she takes in and with whom she will form a lasting relationship. However, this relationship will in fact be "a state of bondage" that "guarantees that possession of her shall continue undisturbed and make her resist new impressions and enticements from the outside" (193). Literally, she will be written upon one time and in a lasting fashion. This writing happens when she gives herself to the man who "takes" her virginity.

This one-time possession and overcoming of the woman's will creates a state of bondage that Freud defines somewhat ironically, with the help of Krafft-Ebing, as a "person's acquiring an unusually high degree of dependence and lack of self-reliance in relation to another person with whom one has a sexual relationship" (193). This bondage runs so deep that the person will sacrifice his or her own self-interest for the other. Some measure of sacrifice is indispensable, Freud says, to the maintenance of civilized marriage and monogamy. The ends justify the means.

Freud points out that for Krafft-Ebing sexual bondage is the result of being in love and having both a weak character *and* unbounded egoism. Unhappy with the seeming contradiction between weakness and strength of character, Freud says the decisive factor is rather the amount of sexual resistance and the modes by which that resistance is overcome. In the emphasis on the "one-time" loss of virginity, the kind of libidinal overhaul desired is a lot to ask of one event. Generalizing, Freud notes that the state of bondage is much more frequent in women than in men, but he adds that it is seen in men much more now than in ancient times. This state of sexual bondage happens in relation to the man's having overcome psychical impotence (something he previously named a universal characteristic of male love) with one woman to whom he will remain subsequently bound.

This brings me to one of my favorite sentences in Freud: "Many strange marriages and not a few tragic events—even some with far-reaching consequences—seem to owe their explanation to this origin" (194). If the libidinal overhaul that Freud cheekily names sexual bondage occurs (especially in the face of extreme inhibition or resistance), it leads to many strange marriages and some tragic events. The wholesale overcoming of resistance is dangerous, which means that the taboo on virginity (or at least the taboo on the attempt to possess the virgin) is a necessary prohibition! At this point, we might ask: How did Freud move from virginity to psychical impotence, to resistance and its overcoming, to consenting to monogamous possession and sexual bondage, and finally to tragic events and tragic marriages?

To put the pieces of this picture of contemporary love life together, Freud returns to virginity as a historical and anthropological question. If one considers the attitude of "primitive" people, they do place a value on virginity. But they value it differently, not emphasizing possession but rather making it taboo. What does this tell us? Freud gets rather fixated on studies that examine what happens when someone must be summoned to rupture the hymen or perform mock-coitus on virgins. He goes through the usual suspects to explain this ritual: the primal fear of blood, the prohibition against murder, sadism, discomfort with menstruation, and the fear or apprehension of anything new, any first time, any occasion for the unexpected or uncanny.

Curiously, when moving from bondage to taboo, Freud slides the word "possession" back in. The sexual bondage first implied—this desire to possess a woman, her sexual memory in the past and in her future—is transformed into the idea that the virgin is literally possessed. She is the possession of some ancestral spirit, which is why the priest and not her mere mortal husband has to rupture her hymen. The difference between possession and possession turns on the question of exclusivity—who possesses her? To whom does she belong? To herself? To her ancestors? To her husband? To her parents?

This brings us to Freud's final point: he says that women, in general, are taboo. They must be kept separate from the men; they are a challenge to men's self-possession, and the barriers of separation need to be firmly in place to mitigate this "generalized dread of women" (198). Freud's brilliance emerges:

> Woman is different from man, forever incomprehensible and mysterious, strange and therefore apparently hostile. The man is afraid of being weakened by the woman, infected with her femininity and of then showing himself incapable. The effect which coitus has of discharging tensions and causing flaccidity may be the prototype of what the man fears; and the realization of the influence which the woman gains over him through sexual intercourse, the consideration she thereby forces from him, may justify the extension of this fear. *In all this there is nothing obsolete, nothing which is not still alive among ourselves.*
>
> (198–99; italics mine)

The question of the virgin's possession comes back in Freud's phrase: "nothing obsolete . . . nothing which is not still alive among ourselves." This shows how easily the woman will possess the man and the living knowledge of this fact, which is what requires women to be taboo.

We have a kind of impasse between wanting to possess the woman, not wanting even to get near her, her possession of him, and her as simply possessed. What else is this besides the eternal war between the sexes and the failure of the sexual relationship? The inability to tolerate separation? Freud suddenly addresses the notion of the "narcissism of minor differences," a process that takes place between the sexes, saying that the greatest hostilities arise in the face of small differences, protecting oneself against feelings of fellowship and love, creating a sensation of strangeness—a first reference to this concept before its infamous characterization of group psychology in the 1921 essay. This narcissism of minor differences underlies "the narcissistic rejection of women by men, which is so mixed up in despising them" (199).

After this statement, Freud seems to want to rein himself in—"we have strayed very far"—and none of this meandering, he claims, helps us with the question of first sexual acts with virgins. There is fear, clearly. But something in this fear or apprehension must be correct, no? There must be some "real" aspect of the apprehension, yes? If it is not simply the man's rejection of love and fellowship with women, then there must be something actually to be dreaded on the side of the woman. What is it?

In one of the essay's strangest paragraphs, Freud says that a woman at climax of sexual satisfaction presses a man to her as an expression of her gratitude and as a gesture of lasting sexual bondage. But, he says, we know "it is by no means the rule that the first occasion of intercourse should lead to this behavior; very frequently it means only disappointment for the woman, who remains cold and unsatisfied" (201). Only with frequent repetition can she find satisfaction, but Freud has observed that this too may not always work, as many women end up in "cheerless and obstinate frigidity" that no tender effort of a husband can overcome. It is this that Freud says we do not sufficiently understand. Of course, many here would interpret that Freud's own masculine bias—his feeling of impotence in the face of women—has caused him to turn away from his own radical diagnosis of misogyny, but even if true in part, we shouldn't simply rush to this conclusion. The paper is strange enough.

It is quite clear, Freud implies, when a woman's dissatisfaction is the result of an insufficiency in the man to overcome his dread, which leads to his psychical impotence. But what is it when it is *her own* resistance that produces perpetual dissatisfaction? We always find this double movement in Freud. The men are easy to understand. He can even diagnose the ills of monogamy and misogyny on the basis of what is easily understood—the tendency to debasement, fear of fellowship with women, fear of her influence, fear of his own psychical impotence. But then there is the question of something *real* on the side of women, something that cannot be reduced to disappointment with men.

Should her resistance not be given its own validity? Freud wonders what to make of the resistance of women themselves. Is the resistance to losing sexual value? Is it intercourse as a narcissistic injury, the destruction of her sense of the integrity of her body? Is it that women are so influenced by their decisions regarding love that to have any sense of their own will they can give themselves only in illicit affairs? Does sexual intercourse assault a woman's pride? Does it, as in the man's case, stem from not wanting to owe a debt of gratitude to men?

Freud points out that we know in psychoanalysis how important the earliest allocations of libido are. The husband is always only a substitute. He is "never the right man" (201). In this depiction of modern love, we have a man who wants to be the only man and a woman for whom this man who wants to be the only man is never the right man. There is always another one, the original. The more powerful this original "psychical" element in a woman's sexual life, the more resistance, Freud says, will be shown by her libido to any upheaval. Bodily possession will overpower her very little, will produce very little effect. She is already possessed by her father and also by her mother (a fact Freud came to later in his work), and she will not tolerate any substitute.

A woman's reactions to this *never the right man* leads Freud to discuss a whole host of archaic feelings aroused by first intercourse or first love, making the taboo on women *reasonable enough*. Freud descends into a series of examples of women's bitter hostility toward men—their desire for revenge, castration, beheading, and the like—and says that when women can't leave a man they have clearly fallen out with, they have not completed their revenge upon him, which keeps them bound to the relationship. The possessed woman must exhaust her sadism—a new twist on the concept of sexual bondage. Second marriages, Freud declares, are often better. The archaic reaction is drained, and women can suddenly be tender. Firsts are terrible, whether you are or wanted to be.

Is this really the *real* in women? Are women full of desires for revenge against their fathers and men who aren't their fathers? Freud is right and wrong in fascinating ways, as he always is when it comes to discussing the Other sex. This essay turns on the word "possession," and this idea—in its two senses—must be overcome by surrendering to bodily upheaval. Whether it is moving the static image into a process, a first-time, actual experience of sexual intercourse into sensual life, the removal of past expectations that brought disappointment into an experience of something new, the removal of fixations on fathers and mothers, or the feeling of dread into a feeling of fellowship, Freud literally describes this as a kind of writing, a writing that only bodily possession can do, this idea of somatic upheaval or, as I call it, *conversion*.

First, we need to consider the concept of conversion in terms of what troubled Freud in the relation between psyche and soma and what he felt was too obscure to understand in conversion symptoms. The "leap into the organic" has often been rendered as the speaking body, something that has been contested in the history of psychoanalytic thought, even against the so-called Lacanians.[1] It is important that the "leap" is not a moment in which the body expresses an idea; it is an activation of old pathways within the organic realm for the purposes of unconscious conflict.[2] What Freud and Breuer are careful to show is not an act of translating an idea through soma, or of expressing this idea somatically, but rather the utilization of already present associations in relation to soma from old pains and injuries to bodily sites of trauma and favored erotogenic zones. This preserves the leap as a leap, past pains as past pains, memories as memories. Psyche is not sutured to soma via an act of assumed symbolization, failed symbolization, or even restored symbolization. Instead, one uses the other in a process of hysterical conversion. In other words, psyche uses the pathways of the body just as the present uses the past.

Conversion holds to the notion of the movement of large quantities of excitation regardless of whether the symptom is bodily. The possibility of bodily upheaval separates itself from mere psychosomatic symptoms and shows the importance of reorganizing a surface that psychoanalysis locates as material, psychical, and corporeal. We neither collapse soma with psyche nor use a problematic causal logic—that is, that the idea or conflict gave rise to a somatic symptom. Indeed, in preserving the distinction between representation and organic processes, the unconscious is given its place as a kind of writing that organizes both the field of representation and the surface of the body together, that is, what we might call the sexual. In fact, without maintaining the separation between psyche and soma in this way, it is precisely the sexual as such that loses its place of prominence, putting either the body and affective processes, or linguistic or psychological representations, forward as primary. This is a war that delineates most trends in psychoanalysis.

The sexual is essentially what saves us, what preserves psyche, and what moves us past the vicissitudes of possession. Possession, as Freud characterizes it, is resistance to the sexual. This is what we see arise as the question of monogamous love in Freud's essay on virginity—how does any of this remain sexual and not degrade into a state of bondage or a war between the sexes? In *Group Psychology and the Analysis of the Ego* ([1921] 1995), Freud refers back to the concept of bondage from "The Taboo on Virginity" in his chapter on love and hypnosis. He places sexual satisfaction and the overvaluation characteristic of love in stark opposition. He does this to highlight the force that binds individuals into a mass and what breaks them apart, even if what they are broken apart into is simply into the sexual loving couple. Love as overvaluation sans sexual desire is linked to sexual bondage and hypnosis because the ego surrenders itself to the object. Hypnosis, like group psychology, utilizes aim-inhibited impulses or, in other words, the lack of sexual satisfaction necessary in the affective tie between leader and follower to sustain this impoverishment of the ego.

What is fascinating and almost counterintuitive is that Freud places continued sexual satisfaction on the side of reality because satisfaction reduces the inclination to overidealize a lover and indiscriminately surrender oneself to the object or give in to the inhibition emanating from a relation to an ideal. Freud writes, "the object has, so to speak, consumed the ego . . . this happens especially easily with love that is unhappy and cannot be satisfied; for in spite of everything each sexual satisfaction always involves a reduction in sexual overvaluation" ([1921] 1995, 113). One is most out of touch with reality when one stays in an unsatisfying sexual relationship, because what purpose can the relationship possibly serve aside from wiping out one's critical sensibilities? Freud famously quotes George Bernard Shaw's "malicious" aphorism that love greatly exaggerates the difference between one woman and another. There is this exaggeration, and then there is the more real question of satisfaction.

I do not believe that Freud is engaging in a wholesale dismissal of love. He simply says that it is a relatively newer development in the history of human civilization, and it is one that should be considered in its ties to mass psychology insofar as mass psychology fosters the splitting of love and desire: "Two people coming together for the purpose of sexual satisfaction, insofar as they seek for solitude, are making a demonstration against the herd instinct, the group feeling. The more they are in love, the more completely they suffice to each other" ([1921] 1995, 140). Turning away from the conundrums of love toward unbridled sex is not what Freud is prescribing—something that he says, in any case, arises in the tendency of groups to throw off the shackles of servitude from time to time and import more regressive psychic elements into group surrender. Sexual love in itself is not the problem, since love is a demonstration against the herd instinct. It is the asexual hypnotic love of leaders that proves the most problematic. The group thrives on the split between love and desire, which nevertheless will be its own undoing.

Uncertain as to the future of either groups or sexual monogamy, there is an urgency in Freud to sense what might be possible in the narrow straights between the demands of object love and sexual desire. Freud suggests that this conundrum is a consequence of the barrier against incest, the necessity for totemic exogamy, which drives a wedge between men's affectionate and sexual feelings. This is a historical event that is inscribed in sexual development in the form of diphasic sexuality. The affectionate always has links to the family and the group, while sexuality is on the side of breaking away (the charge of adolescence).

> Even in a person who has in other respects become absorbed in a group, the directly sexual impulsions preserve a little of his individual activity. If they become too strong they disintegrate every group formation ... falling in love has often driven even priests to leave the church. In the same way love for women breaks through group ties of race, of national divisions, and of social class systems, and it thus produces important effects as a factor in civilization.
>
> ([1921] 1995, 141)

Sexual love of women is asocial.[3] It transcends the ties of any group. This would be true in heterosexuality, if in fact the man sexually loved a woman rather than simply repudiating her. This would also be true in homosexuality, either by women or by men, when the desire is for women, loosely defined. Strange how dangerous women keep proving to be.

Freud points out that this asociality is also true for neurosis, which has the same "disintegrating effect" (142). Where there is group formation, there is less neurosis—which may temporarily disappear. One might turn this into a kind of therapeutic enterprise: this is the strategy of any cult or guru or even psychoanalytic sect, as "all the ties that bind people to mystico-religious or philosophico-religious sects and communities are expressions of crooked cures of all kinds of neuroses" (142). While many may not regret the disappearance of religious illusions from the civilized world, Freud says that we must nevertheless admit that they are a powerful shield against the dangers of neurosis.

In the neurotics' exile from the group mind, they create their own mythological universe—"he creates his own world of imagination for himself, his own religion, his own system of delusions, and thus recapitulates the institutions of humanity in a distorted way which is clear evidence of the dominating part played by the directly sexual impulsions" (142). Like the sexual love of women, neurosis saves us from the group in its contortions and parodies of the institutions of humanity. In *Totem and Taboo* ([1913b] 1995), the same dilemma between the institutions of humanity and the private realm of neurosis is famously alluded to by Freud in his comparison of hysteria and art, obsessional neurosis and religion, and paranoia and philosophy.

What, then, would not be a "crooked cure"? Or, what conversion is possible that isn't a conversion into mass psychology? Or, perhaps better, what, if anything, can be done with a sexuality that cannot unite men like self-preservation does and that is essentially a private affair? Freud laments that neurosis is a flight from reality into a world of wishful fantasy, yet there is something more real in the distortions of human culture found in the dream life and symptom formations of neurosis. Are these "distortions" not what are held onto against what is "dissatisfying" in reality?

It is here where I think we are close to the point of conversion that we located in hysteria. Freud seems to suggest this when he says that "the real world, which is avoided in this way by neurotics, is under the sway of human society and of the institutions collectively created by it" ([1913b] 1995, 74). While many have read this as a statement about the flight of neurotics from the community of men, it can perhaps be read as insinuating that the real world is both avoided by neurotics *and* held captive by human institutions. There is a question of how to touch this real. How do we find it if not by overcoming the avoidance and inhibitions of the neurotics, who are the ones who have withdrawn from the collective that holds it captive? Freud ends *Group Psychology* by indicating that neuroses are "extraordinarily rich in content, for they embrace *all possible* relations between the ego and the object" ([1921] 1995, 143; italics mine).

Neurosis is a means of knotting the ego, ego-ideal, and the object through some new form of identification. The main unanswered question in *Group Psychology*—"can there be no identification when the object is retained?"—seems to ask what might be discovered within, not outside of, neurosis. This question concerning the forms of identification in Freud always slips into a discussion of melancholia, for what is melancholia but this conundrum of giving up the object or identifying with it? At the most extreme end, melancholia is the solution of identifying with the object, which is retained as rejected. You keep it by rejecting it internally, holding onto it in an identification with the object as lost—a conundrum of separation if there ever was one. The necessity to exhaust rage against the lost object is similar to that of the women in "The Taboo on Virginity." The body is searching for a point of upheaval and reconfiguration.

Further, a kind of truthfulness about the "real world" also makes its appearance in melancholia's bluntness about the ephemerality of life and the flaws of humanity. As Freud put it, "we only wonder why a man has to be ill before he can be accessible to a truth of this kind" ([1917a] 1995, 246–47). This truthfulness about the real world is linked to a question of hysteria as what is scotomized, including women's apprehension of a failure inherent in men (or simply others) and what civilization requires of men at the expense of loving women (what Freud called the anhedonia in men that makes women hysterical in marriage). Yet there is something beyond all this, or in addition to it, that Freud is searching for—something one might call the real impossibility of sexuality that neurosis aims to resolve without abandoning sexual love or sexual satisfaction and without turning away from "women." Again, I want to name this as conversion, which gives a particular reading of the work required by mourning.

When describing the conundrums of conscience, especially in melancholic guilt, Freud says that "in the blindness of love remorselessness is carried to the pitch of a crime" ([1921] 1995, 113), which is like a manic triumph over melancholia. This remorselessness occurs when the differentiating gradations between the ego-ideal and the ego collapses. The solution is momentary, false, a manic rationalization, but nevertheless this criminal remorselessness harbors within it a possible solution in sexual object love. The gap between the ego and ego-ideal is where the melancholic slaughters him- or herself and where neurosis springs forward. What could the remorselessness of love look like if it wasn't simply a denial of mourning or the temptation to abandon all sense of reality? What does remorselessness have to do with a different kind of identification, one that includes the possibility of loss?

We saw that the malaise of civilized life is countered by the psychoanalytic cure, which pushes back against the costs of civilized morality, making psychoanalysis asocial, like the love of women and neurosis more generally. Conversion is the solution insofar as it reclaims the pleasure that civilization has extracted from each of us. The hysteric forces her desire into the outside world in the act of creating an object through which she can find some new satisfaction. She has to do this without the action resulting in psychosis, hysterical hallucinatory confusion, or a lapse back into archaic possession or anhedonia.

The ill-defined term "sublimation" hovers in the background. The one qualification of sublimation that Freud ventured was that while it leaves repression intact, it manages to bypass it economically, bringing with it a full experience of satisfaction. It overcomes resistance that has used the depletion of satisfaction to its own ends, pushing back against the costs of civilized sexual morality. How could this not be remorseless? The gap between one's aptitude in relation to the world and one's ideal is where the neurotic person usually founders, where the powers of sublimation evade the possible solutions at hand.

This gap closes in the moment of sublimation's experienced pleasure, where the externalization of a desire can be reinternalized. Closing this gap, even if only for a moment, requires its own pitch, its own criminal remorselessness, and perhaps blindness as well. The work is not about the construction of the object as lost, for conversion here takes on a slightly different valence, moving from the loss of the object to the loss and rediscovery of libido. This is what must be constructed, returning to us what has been split off and remains threatened from the side of civilization. This work is more on the side of the body than on the object, and it requires a remorselessness from both the patient and the analyst.[4]

As I see it, the problem is that love relations are too precarious when faced with such a great psychical necessity. This is what Freud means when he considers pessimistically the overcoming of sexual bondage, the dread of women, psychical impotence, and the disappointments and difficulties of erotic life. The crooked cure by one human institution or another is a great lure. There is also the danger of lapsing into a kind of Reichean orgone theory and getting lost in the search for the perfect cancer-curing orgasm. Freud seems only to have faith in sublimation as a creative endeavor, though the problem, he said, is that it was only available to a select few and requires the capacity to tolerate long periods of frustration and waiting. Rather than love or work, perhaps what we should locate here is a question of the psychoanalytic cure.

I want to think psychoanalytic work as writing from the place of a loss or knot in one's libido, this point-for-point encounter between the more hysterical analysand and her analyst. It has more possibility for creating some new configuration because, at the very least, the analyst knows how to make him- or herself the object of love without a promise and without a body, allowing him- or herself to become an object that you, the patient, inscribe from the outside in, disappearing so that what is written is yours. The analyst is the one who knows how to break language, not make it, so these lines intensify, to the point of something dire, the force of conversion: because the analyst is the one who can hear the appeal, the elegant articulation of a symptom, using this point to push the contradictions in the appeal to love, kicking back against nihilism, melancholia, love as consumerism, disappointment, and finally (our biggest enemy) inhibition, since it always leads to violence.

Maybe it is not a question of first intercourse, or even of first marriages, good marriages, or better illusions or collective fictions, but simply a question of first analyses—what analysis can make possible, especially when it makes room for remorselessness in all its melancholic and drive-ridden vicissitudes. The archaic reactions, exhausting themselves there, can open onto what Freud called the somatic preserve, the inexhaustible reserve in the body. And isn't this simply another name for the transference to the psychoanalyst, here not simply the midwife but the one who assumes the role of *never the right man*? This *never the right man* psychoanalyst is the only one able to take on a patient in the name of conversion.

V

I AM NOT A MUSE

"Danton, your lips have eyes": That is not a "modern metaphor," that is knowledge, from afar, concerning [visionary] knowledge of a mouth.

—PAUL CELAN, *THE MERIDIAN: FINAL VERSION—DRAFTS—MATERIALS*

I AM NOT A MUSE

If we give this virgin a voice, what would she say? Let us begin with returning to her other Freudian name: the hysteric! Speak this name, and they almost immediately seem to ask: "Where is she? Where has she gone?" As if a question of presence or the evocation of the absence of a person is something that should be held by a vigilant gaze. Sadly, that's just the psychoanalysts muttering to themselves, an equally questionable clan with their own mumbled troubles—"Where are we?" "Are we on our way out?" "Who even wants us anymore?" These questions are so difficult because they seem so obvious, because they seem like they deserve a simple answer, where all the anxiety about disappearance, elusiveness, and ambiguity is concealed in this demand. Does the hysteric even want to be found by this anxious analyst?

In *Civilization and Its Discontents* ([1930] 1995), Freud notes that "writing to begin with was the voice of the absent" (49). We write only because we or another has been lost. He writes this in a text that declares that he doesn't care if civilization disappears, as if then—finally—we can catch up with writing, catch up with an unconscious that was the essence of absence writ. It is not up to me, Freud says, to judge the value of civilization. Perhaps Eros will win. Perhaps the death drive, silent and still, will conquer all. We should be prepared to lose everything. Contrast this sentiment with his famous statement about the finding of an object always being a refinding. If the hysteric is disappearing as a clinical entity, if the particular obsession is with her place, perhaps we could apply this Freudian logic and ask what it would mean not to care if she disappeared. What might letting her write this voice of absence bring on a profession that finds its birthright with her?

There is something to be learned from the disappearance of the hysteric and her new name, which labels woman not as an entity—historical, heroic, or pathologized—but rather as a social question: *conversion disorder*. What does hysteria mean when her intractable irrelevance is no longer the result of hatred, radical suppression, or even indifference; when the engines of fascination have exhausted themselves, and we approach something on the order of radical erasure? We no longer even know what the word "hysteria" means, yet it is part of a common lexicon, an adjective, seamless with the blah blah blah of everyday chatter. She is everywhere and nowhere, as if the disorder had spread so much it has become invisible.

"Hysteria" is part of the name of an old New York experimental theater whose productions feel dated. It is also the name of a new pilot TV show that is part graduate-school lecture on hysteria from witches to boarding schools and part *Law and Order*/medical-mystery serial television. It is something Lacanians talk about with a special aura (the hysteric!), which implies some kind of rarified knowledge, despite the fact that it is about what cannot be known. Being hysterical is now equivalent to the idea of being really emotional, excessively emotional, which can also be seen as empty of anything. It could be epitomized by the emoticon in a text message.

You don't ask about it. It's just there. Someone crying. Someone pulling at their hair, or with an exaggerated expression on their face, cheeks turning red, with hearts for eyes, sweating or surprised. Do emoticons clarify what is being said, or are they a surplus, distracting or overturning what is written? Even Munch's scream is now an emoticon: awash, excessive, but silent. Content without content, like women on reality TV who only talk about what it means to be a woman by screaming or talking really fast or being fascinated by one another's bodies. TV is an empire of women who play the hysteric when it suits them. Hysteria is reduced to a look or a gesture or to pure performativity.

The word has no weight. Weightless, it is unburdened from history. Excessive and then erased; monumental, then subdivided and dismantled. Mantled and dismantled in a single movement. Perhaps that's the point. The spreading surface of hysteria is carried along by the currents of history, truer than any content could ever be, could ever have been. And the two ends of the circle of the story of hysteria meet at this point X. Hysteria realizes itself in this act of erasure, in the gathering and dispersal of desire. Desire is rendered as pure form and formal movement, set adrift, creating in its wake a demand for this drift and a counterdemand set against it. Hysteria's disappearing act—showing us the formal characteristics of the drive, the reliance on a game of presence and absence, and the potential instigation of a desire that spreads outward, that refuses to stay still, locked into any one set of meanings.

We might wonder about her place in this. We might wonder if, in orchestrating her disappearance, she has found a way to exist a little more easily outside of any diagnostic demands. Perhaps this is always where she felt destined to go, while *we* imagine some abuse of a barbaric present, the travesty of the gender war of contemporary medicine, which erases hysteria from history in an act of violence. The good doctor raises his hand and vies for securing her place. There is still so much to be said about the hysteric! Let us not stop here! Yet, from another angle of history, these doctors were always a burden for the hysteric. Whether she was on a pedestal, performing for them, or locked away in a sanatorium (too much for them), it was a lot to live up to. Perhaps now, as history dissolves into this unnamable and formally beautiful point X, the hysteric will finally belong to no one. Conversion disorder is the equivalent to her saying: "I have nothing to do with you. I am not a muse."

I often forget that the word "hysteria" also suggests amusement, laughter, comedy—another important yet sedimented iteration in common usage. That's hysterical! It's hysterical! I like this meaning! It suggests the world has recognized that there is something important about humor and the hysteric. As if hysteria flipped into its other more manic self, evoked by the supposedly inappropriate giggling that annoyed so many of the doctors early on. And what did they say about this giggling?—that it was out of step with what she was saying, that it was defensive, sexual, seductive, the result of too much internal tension. That it was, well, hysterical. What a tautology! She's hysterical because she's hysterical.

What kind of humor is hysterical? Nonsense seems right. There is something important about the disappearance of sense, the slide toward nonsense, striving toward the limit of sense—what is idiotic in trying to make sense of anything. Laughter is the best punctuation. It requires nothing more. There is nothing to add to the senselessness of existence, or, rather, adding anything violates an already violent loss of meaning that haunts us all. I'm always relieved when I am absolved of the demand to make sense with a patient in session, which happens when a patient laughs, when they've said something absolutely hysterical. Afterward, no one has to say anything else; the silence is not imposed by either of us. Hysteria disappears in what is hysterical.

HER MAJESTY THE ABSURD

The poet Paul Celan has another name for this vanishing point embodied by hysteria. He calls it the majesty of the absurd. This phrase condenses the disappearing point in language with the moment of encounter, something Celan also names *the poem* in his "Meridian Speech," given when he received the Buchner Prize in 1960. It is a breathtakingly beautiful piece of writing, and it has been read by scholars as a statement about Celan's vision of poetry and aesthetics more generally. Poetic absurdity is announced for him by female figures, particularly by Lucile in Buchner's "Danton's Death."

For Celan, the majesty of the absurd often sounds like something else, like Lucille's words on the gallows during the French Revolution, "long live the king." But, he warns us, "it is not what it seems," especially when it seems like allegiance to an "ancien régime," to some worship of kings, to some yesterday worth preserving (Celan 2011, 13). Lucille is not invested in revolution, monarchy, cutting off heads, or being a martyr. She is interested in what bespeaks the presence of human beings. Her words open a moment of encounter.

She repeats your words back to you—"long live the king!"—and in this repetition, her king is always already an absurdity, a hysterical absurdity that she announces at the moment of their retaliation and her disappearance. "And this," Celan says, "has to do only indirectly with the—not to be underestimated—difficulties of word choice, the faster fall of syntax or the more lucid sense for ellipses" (8). In speaking this majesty of the absurd, Celan insists that she is like the poem itself. She stands her ground and shows the tendency toward silence, calling and pulling herself back from an "already no more" into an "always still." "This always-still can only be a speaking. But not just language as such, nor presumably, just verbal 'analogy' either. But language actualized, set free under the sign of radical individuation that at the same time, however, remains mindful of the borders language draws and the possibilities language opens up for it" (9).

Celan here teaches us about hysteria—the special dialect that hysteria engenders—which repeats not merely to mock but to change and wrest something free in language, from language. One might call this conversion. The hysterical proclamation is not an attempt to solidify a yesteryear but to change the nature of dialogue itself. It is for this reason that Lacan turned to the hysterics in his 1977 essay "Propos sur l'hystérie":

> Where have they gone, the hysterics of yesteryear, those wonderful women, the Anna O.s, or the Emmy von N.s . . . ? They not only played a certain role, certainly a social role, but when Freud started to listen to them, it was they who allowed for the birth of psychoanalysis. By listening to them Freud inaugurated an entirely new mode of human relations. What has replaced the hysterical symptoms of yesteryear? Has hysteria not been displaced to the social field?
>
> (Lacan 1977, 5)

The hysteric's discourse operates by constantly posing a question, and in so doing she plays an important social role. She desires "a new mode of human relations."

In light of Celan's "Meridian Speech," I'd like to say that I'm tired of the definition of hysteria as a pathological relationship to masters and fathers, as a conflict around castration and the phallus, male and female power dynamics, and what have you. If conversion disorder speaks to a desire for another order of human relations in a way that hysteria no longer can, then I celebrate the disappearance of the term. Conversion picks up where hysteria left off and radicalizes the encounter with psychoanalysis.

Celan says that this moment takes our breath away, makes the medusa heads shrink and the engines break down, for a moment. And in that moment when something falls out, shrivels, and runs down, it is enough. The throne is finally seen for what it is: empty. This happens at this point of conversion. The hysteric waits for this *enough*. Perhaps she alone knows what is enough. I realize this is absurd to suggest—the hysteric knows what is enough? Isn't she the one who is the most attached to dissatisfaction? The answer is unreservedly: no. Her dissatisfaction serves her in the search for what is, finally, enough, and enough to reinvent.

One of the great ironies of psychoanalysis is that it is born from an encounter with the hysteric and fears dying when she disappears. Yet Freud mostly gave up writing on women after Dora. We have two failed countercases: the female homosexual whom he referred for treatment to someone else and his case of paranoia running counter to the disease, a woman he saw twice in consultation. Most of Freud's writings on women, as I have said, are fraught with exasperation, while the hysterics chase what Freud called, in *Civilization and Its Discontents*, their claim on love. Love, Freud states with disdain, was a difficult and unwieldy basket to put all their eggs in, compared to, say, gardening or theoretical research.[1]

Lacan, on the other hand, wanted to talk about women. His first clinical works centered on psychotic women and the shudder they sent through the homes of the bourgeois French family. The surrealists found a parable in his cases because they spoke to the formal beauty of their art, a practice of paranoiac critique and a revolution in our sense of reality. Yet, when one looks at Lacan's body of work, he spoke more about his hatred of modern-day analysis, paranoia, and obsessionality, maybe fetishism and the phallus, more than he ever did about the hysteric. He's best when he becomes hysterical and approaches her there, but these moments are rare.

When Lacan does address the hysteric, these are powerful moments in his seminar. Dora remains a model for the obstacles to and possibilities of a uniquely psychoanalytic cure. In Lacan's reading, he shows how Freud's dialectical synthesis of her unfolding case reveals a logical coherence equal to the best mathematical formulae. A good analyst will see every point of stagnation in a case reflected in his own deafness—his own biases and imaginary expectations—particularly as they stem from the encounter with women. Only hysteria seems to be able really to teach psychoanalysts how to listen. What does the hysteric want? Lacan answers: "You'll see!"

Lacan turns to Freud's countertransference to women, pointing to the opening dream of Freud's *Traumdeutung*, which is centered on the hysterical woman Irma, who hides a multitude of hysterics beneath her image. Freud's dream of Irma's injection should be read in assemblage: Lacan pointing to Freud's deepening hysteria in the dream book, the acephalic self-amputation of Freud, the prehistoric voice from beyond, the enigmatic formula for desire that says everything and nothing, the writing on the wall, the dream that simply asks that it be acknowledged as written, a punctum of meaning that is also the degeneration of sense, a nonsense word that is a cipher for desire, the desire for desire, ad infinitum. Here, Freud disappears behind the wish, the navel of the dream, and the formula for psychoanalysis appears in bold print before him: the dream is a wish and nothing more. This wish has to be written into existence.

Think also of Lacan's use in his seminar from 1961, *Transference*, of Claudel's terrifyingly strange female figures—Sygne, Lumyir, Pensée—cloaked in a supposedly Catholic drama by a figure more or less forgotten. Lacan says about the trilogy's final figure, Pensée, the blind girl:

> The mysterious power of the dialogue which takes place between Pensée and Orian . . . this mysterious admission with which this dialog ends: "I am blind" has, just by itself, the force of an "I love you" because it avoids any awareness in the other of the "I love you" being said, in order to go straight and place itself in him as a word. Who could say: "I am blind" except from where the word creates the night? Who, in hearing it, would not feel coming to birth in himself this depth of night?
>
> (Lacan 2016, 262)

Here, Lacan does not speak about counterfeit fathers, impotent men, or symptoms passed down between the generations. Even women with their bodily symptoms and will to sacrifice can be eclipsed by the force of a word, a word taken into the body and, like a hysterical pregnancy, feeling its coming to birth, this dawning of a depth of night. How marvelous that is! And how difficult! I am blind. I am burning. I am what I am. I love you.

These moments that Lacan points out in Freud concern the conversion that evokes an enough: "What Claudel means by the blind Pensée is that *it is enough* that the soul should close its eyes to the world in order to be able to be that which the world lacks . . . the most desirable object in the world" (262). We need to close our eyes to the world in order to be what the world lacks, and in this we become the most desirable object in the world, which isn't a virtue, because no one wants to get too close. But to be this object is not to bemoan what we imagine is lacking but instead to disappear in hysteria.

HOW TO DISAPPEAR

Every day in my practice I hear something of the vicissitudes of this disappearing act within a moment of conversion. How this moment of vanishing arises is usually one the most powerful moments in the treatment; it is where the analyst, amid this fevered discourse, is forced to find her place. Ilene comes in to see me. She is quite young but has an aura of age. She is dressed like a techno goddess: brightly colored hair, platform shoes, lace, leather, black eyeliner, a large choker on her neck that elongates it like those women from a distant tribe—old and futuristic at once. She called just before her mother died, anticipating her death, saying she thought it would be good to mourn with the help of an analyst. I couldn't see her for a couple of months. She said with determination that her mother would probably be dead and she would be ready then. She wasn't looking for a replacement. She wanted to get back to herself. Her mother had been ill for a very long time.

What I would find out upon meeting Ilene was that her mother was first diagnosed with a rare disease when she was seven but had survived for twenty years after her first diagnosis, through three surgeries, until her final decline, which lasted about two years. After her first collapse, her mother couldn't drive again for fear of seizures. The majority of Ilene's care fell to her rather melancholic father and her grandmother, who was all too happy to have another child to look after. Ilene was close to her mother, and when she was older—like a little mother herself—she looked after her entire family, especially her father, whose life was a shrine to his wife.

The issue that surfaced immediately with Ilene was a recurrent sense she had of being in her body but paralyzed, unable to move, looking out from inside of her eyes and lacking the power of action. Sometimes there was a mood to this inner space, sadness or elation, nostalgia or calm; the air may have a temperature, cold or warm, or be colored, blue or green or crimson or black and white. It was in sensing and visualizing this mood that the paralysis would lift; a strange work with and against dissociation, a daydreamer of Freud's yesteryear.

Ilene created worlds based on these feelings, worlds she brought to life not only on her flesh or in her appearance but in her music, art, and writing, where she enjoyed early success—a success tinged with a veneer of guilt in relation to her sick and dying mother. When not in this place, she felt like she was looking at herself from the outside: self-critical, perfectionistic, the harangue of plans, plans, plans for her future unrealized self. There was a deep sense of urgency as opposed to the languor of wishful thinking.

I wondered about this dissociation and her mother's ill body. I imagined her identification with the mother, who had seizures, and her sense of everything that her mother would not get to do or be. Ilene was safe on the inside, lost on the outside. Or is it the other way around? Inside there is a world of feeling and sensation, electric but passive. Outside, all eyes, all logos—the cruel certainty of a world of potential action and control. One being, the other doing and having.

Surprisingly, it wasn't this sick mother like a saint but in fact the other mother, her grandmother, who came to the fore in the beginning of analysis. I'll hear about the mother sometime in the future. The grandmother had tended to this child in her mother's absence and made her into a repository for all her stifled wishes. One mother that doesn't wish, another that is pure wish. Ilene absorbed this grandmother's love to the point of mortification, locked into obsessional symptoms until adolescence when—in a moment of impulse and impetuousness—she went and told her mother of her troubled relationship with her grandmother. She found herself in the midst of a startling energy aimed at separation—something that seems to leave so many patients once the disappointments of adult life settle in. She broke away from her grandmother at full steam. Never again! Her hair would be her hair; her body would be her body; she would do with it what she liked. She would make *her* daydreams come to life. She would be a living, breathing mood board and not the passive object for the other mother or any mother, for that matter. Mourning began with this first act of separation, which was worn on the outside like a gothic princess.

But her mother's death and a change in her career eventually broke apart this carefully constructed separateness, jettisoning these previous gains. And it is this that brought her to analysis. Her work in psychoanalysis would be the same work she had built as a young girl, work centered on a question of separation and the vicissitudes of being an object for another.

All of her first dreams in analysis entail her losing her passport or needing a new one. I'm not sure if I'm her travel agent or homeland security or border control. I wonder what it is that we have to refind or reissue, and I find myself worrying about losing the vitality of this way of being that she found and used so well, the energy of first solutions, of actively lived separations. Why do so many patients lose these gains in adult life? I suppose that's what Freud means about being neurotic only after puberty, after this total overhaul of sexual life takes place. I'm also sure that the sedimentations of the superego are also to blame once the ego-ideal collapses into the easily reversible figure of counteridentifications.

Ilene develops a new costume in analysis. It involves doubled eyes—the ones you paint on your eyelids so that even when you close your eyes to the world around you, no one will know you are asleep. You can keep false vigilance. "This way I can look inward with ease," she said to me, "a kind of optical illusion or illusion with optics . . . and then I had this feeling of the 1960s mod girls, always dancing, in go-go boots. I will be dancing on the inside. The color palate is black and white with pinks and green." Double eyes, go-go. I go. This is not only her first passport in the analysis; it is her first means of transport, which has the closest of links to ecstasy, to the power of conversion, like movement stirring in a body that allows her to claim it as hers and hers alone. All you need is double vision: I look at you from the place where I no longer see myself.

Vanessa comes. In her first dream, her mouth is full of gum. How many patients have dreamed of having gum stuck in their mouth? I think about chewing gum at school and all the gum under desks. Something about the oral object. Do you let yourself touch it in the place where it accumulates? Vanessa's dream about gum evokes a Polish folk song from childhood that went something like "sour in, sour out, sour mouth, sauerkraut." Her grandmother would dunk her underwater in the pool when she said sauerkraut—the action having something to do with the pickling of cabbage. The dimension of orality is so intense in the little pool game—playing at being the oral object taken in and spit out, preserved or discarded.

A week later, she dreams of having a family with a woman but suddenly has to leave to kill a man and make chop suey with his organs for dinner. Funny. At the time, she had been talking about how she ended up in a lesbian community, dating a woman who made her forswear men, who talked about being abused and the necessity of protecting one another from male violence. An easy repetition of her role with her mother and sister, but that's not the point. The point is rather that she does her homework, and she goes to see for herself. She touches the object where it is expected. She betrayed this little clan's imperative and started dating men. "You touch men's penises!" She was cut off from them, and she's been sad ever since. How can you not go see for yourself? Is this really what is in and what is out?

As the analysis has progressed, it feels as if her song is translated into a means of framing her dreams, which have this uncanny quality of finding herself on a stage, then exiting the scene, zooming out into a sweeping overhead panoramic shoot. In/out. "I bumped into something," she says to me in a session, "over the weekend . . . and I'm feeling a little lighter." She rode her bike at night through the area haunted by her former lover, passing every apartment they lived in or used to frequent, and then she found her way to a movie set, where she was acting in a scene. She felt good about her work. "Both were me and neither was me."

By finding herself in the act of reversing the script of her dreams, from out (the panorama) to in (the scene), she bumped into something. She couldn't say what. Only that she felt better, lighter. This uncanny dramatization and reversal seemed to relieve a sense of heaviness she had been living with. I remember a quotation from Celan—"high art is a dream of great magic, the state of levitation. With it I saw the power of heaviness end" (2011, 97). But, as is usually the case, I was prematurely relieved. The next week, she comes in and tells me she blacked out over the weekend. I feel dismayed. It was inevitable that she would test the other side—that she would have to become the bump in the night.

Julie bangs her forearms until they are bruised. She describes scenes with her mother, who seems unusually fixated on her body, which is either too fat or too sexy—hard to tell. It is also hard for her to hear how insecure her mother is in the face of this daughter who has done remarkably well for herself. Why her forearms? Not sure yet. I remember a song from my childhood that described where you could put your arms at the dinner table: never your elbows, sometimes your forearms, always your wrists. Never, sometimes, always. It's a song between mothers and daughters. The sometimes of forearms was more interesting to me than the always or never. When?

Julie describes a particularly vicious scene with her mother when going to visit her father in the hospital who suddenly fell ill. Her mother tells her that she has to drive with the windows open because her feet smell so bad. There is a long story about her tennis shoes being shuffled around between these two women, putting them in the washing machine, putting them in the back seat of the car—the shoes, the feet, the smell. "I'm not sitting here trapped with the smell of your feet," the mother says to the daughter. The daughter bangs her forearms on the dashboard of the car and tells her mother that she isn't the only one suffering, literalizing her mother's blows. Her mother keeps saying, as she does, "you think I'm stupid, you think I'm uneducated."

In session, right as she says this, Julie suddenly begins to talk about how she realizes how alone she is. Her father may never speak again. Her mother... well, she thought maybe this would have brought them together. She describes the pain in her as dim, dull... I hear stupid. I hear her mother's stupid taken in. I repeat the "dim" and "dull" back to her. I make stupid remarks about this mother getting inside of her. She looks at me coyly, with some pity, and says, "everything you say makes sense, especially when you lay it out like this... but it's so absolutely prehistoric. It's not in me. It is me."

I smile and remember that sometimes she relishes telling me how stupid some white women are. I think about how calmly she smiles while telling me the most horrific things. I think about the word "prehistoric" and jokes about how stupid dinosaurs were supposed to be. I think about extinction. I think about the contradiction of dull pain. I think about the stupidity of feeling hurt by another person. How stupid we all are! I wonder if there is another way to disappear than into this stupid pain. Trauma that evacuates all knowledge. Maybe she's right. This is our extinction.

Whenever Martin comes into the room, he throws himself onto the couch, then he gets up and grabs a handful of tissues, wipes the sweat off his brow, and lies back down again, wanting to show me the new emanation of his rash, also, oddly, usually on his forearms. He gestures theatrically, touching his neck and putting his hand to his head; he takes his glasses on and off, usually saying nothing for the first ten minutes of a session. He reminds me of women in 1920s Hollywood films when they would swoon or faint or collapse. He tells me one day that his shoelaces are always undone and hurries to tie his shoes. People, he says, think he's unprofessional. I ask why he doesn't get shoes without laces, and he looks at me, disgruntled, and says, "they aren't professional looking." Of course! I smile at the absurdity of our exchange, my stupid question.

The point is and always has been a question of "the professional." When it comes to being a professional, you can't win. He directs his proverb at me with vehemence sometimes. One day, he talks about calling his mother after every doctor's appointment—of which he has many; it's almost a full-time career—and I suggest that maybe he might not. "How is that psychoanalytic?" he asks me. I think to myself that one day I'll have to explain to him that I've stopped knowing what in the world "psychoanalytic" means, which doesn't mean I know whether suggesting something overtly—or not—is psychoanalytic. It simply doesn't tell you where the dividing line is.

In a world where everything including psychoanalysis is being professionalized, Martin teaches me something, for he was at one point the consummate professional. Is it unprofessional if you have a constantly bleeding colon? If you have to leave work to go to a doctor's appointment? It's not under his control after all, unlike schedules and emails and to-do lists. What about undone shoelaces? Should that be under his control as well? What control does the psychoanalyst exert? What does professional psychoanalysis tell us about being a professional? Martin's question about the professional is profound: what part of you is your profession? Can your profession be something you do but not who you are in the logic of identification? Doesn't identification mean that you have to be your profession, hence the word "professional"? Can one even speak of *having* a profession rather than *being* it at this point in history?

Every hysteric will tell you about how much they hate soldering their being and their body to their work. They will tell you about the suffocation and about a sense of pure revolt. Like Martin, she points to something we are all beginning to feel about the hidden violence of this new bureaucratic universe, of this new way of being as working, a world of work without any dividing lines. This isn't all of Martin, thank god. There is another passion of his: theater. I think about how theater—drama—is really antiprofessional professionalism. Everyone in theater I've ever met is dead serious while they respect that nothing happens because order has been imposed. Rather, things happen because chaos is allowed to reign, setting the stage in an amazing game of pure repetition that exhausts itself. And theater is about repetition. The violence of repetition. A game of improvisation for the centuries.

Theater, for Martin, manages to take what cuts you to the core in human interchange and dramatizes it—creating aesthetic distance through distillation and exaggeration—so that a lesson can be learned or so that something can be heard. Theater is as much about what is said as what is not said, as well as what is done, often brutally, between loving partners. Nothing is more human than theater, and nothing is more theatrical than humanity. Theater makes you see the world from the outside. Separate from it. From the inside, one lives in the threat of sheer violence or its covering over. I think to myself with Martin that I should know this as a psychoanalyst. Oedipus at Colonus. Outside the city. I hope theater wins and not Martin's colon. This gift he has for the unprofessed. While I put my hopes on this gift, this other profession, Martin confirms every appointment with me by email once, sometimes twice.

Eve is interested in cooking. She knows many recipes by heart, and she tells me about them. She's even started to bring some spices for me to smell, curious what I will or won't like. She'd like to find the coordinates of the flavors I like. I imagine that she's making a chart. Jamieson likes turmeric and doesn't like anise; she might like celery seed. She likes celery seed, but only when it contains a note of cinnamon. She seems to be composing my makeup, one that is somehow not all simply fantasy. I wonder if this is something I should allow. Should I let her get this close to me with something so primordial? I suddenly can't remember if it's the nose or the ear that can't close. You can pinch your nose, but you can also cover your ears. I wonder what feels more invasive, sound or smell. I'd better shut my mouth!

Eve is one of those patients that begins a treatment by telling you about their horrific psychiatric history—hospitalizations, combinations of drugs started at such a young age, endless diagnoses, some good therapy that is somehow still unresolved, and some really, really, terrible therapy. "Depressed" is a word she likes to use a lot, as if it is a cipher for something confusing to her about her future, something melancholic that drains the future of an image. She doesn't feel herself with anyone. She doesn't like the awkwardness of having to get to know anyone. It raises a question about this *herself*, but the point is that her awkwardness meets a general awkwardness in human relationships, and that seems pointless to her, nearly impossible. The realm of the sensory is so much more direct, clear—like disgust and excitement.

She tells me that she first tried to kill herself when she was ten years old by eating something she found in her kitchen whose bottle was light pink but labeled toxic. Such a strange contrast between this childlike object and the deadly index. Hysteria as the contradiction of this object as *pharmakon*: what is a cure is always also poison, what is poison is also a cure. When she was going through puberty and was faced with giving up the toys of childhood, she walked through the mall and encountered a scent in a candy store—it was mostly composed of grapefruit, but there was the smell of plastic in it, she tells me, and it was fleshy-pink colored. She had to have it. It smelled and looked like the dolls she was supposed to leave behind when she became a grown-up girl. "I'll eat it," she thought to herself, along with, "how did they get it so right?" Especially when everything else feels so wrong. And it was. She only recently stopped compulsively snacking on this candy.

The question of what can be memorialized and so marked as lost only happens through food. All else is painfully awkward. Speaking is repulsive, and the connections that must be sought are somehow too hard, take too long, are too ambiguous. "With aromatic cooking," she tells me, "it's about an imagined future identity . . . it tells me who I can or want to imagine myself to be, at a certain moment, at a particular time, without having to say it, without perhaps even having to know anything about it." Femininity is fragrant and emanates from the future. The persistent question about a future female self happens without even knowing it. This is the way to open up a dull and disappointing present.

As her analyst, I have to say, I feel disappointing to her already. I know she prefers looking at me, the smell of my office, its décor, my facial gestures, to anything I end up saying, which falls utterly flat, which tries to predict too much for someone wed to futurity, even when it means the present collapses (which it does daily). I think of her neglected writing, her neglected passions and possibilities, and I wonder if I'm filling up some kind of hole, like so many figures in the past, or if I'm something that will come to her from the future. If only I could find a way for my words to match this disjointed temporality. The question—hearing this desire—is a start, or could be.

Every one of these patients is a hysteric, perched at a particularly hysterical moment of their analysis. This is also a way of saying that not one of them is a hysteric really, for it's about a certain configuration that emerges in analysis. I don't want to turn my patients into muses, in which case I would locate myself in a relation of worship or hate or fascination. To attempt to negate this possibility provides a certain degree of comfort. I am not a muse either. We need to listen to something else, in some other way—this something that I am calling "conversion disorder." In it there is a certain danger; it is a danger of joining these patients too much here, a joining that always feels like falling asleep, too much in the body.

The precarity of walking this line—trying to separate amusement from pathos, to search for what will keep me awake—is a better line to walk than the veneration or hatred of hysteria. It's not an easy task, but I've learned better how to walk this line *from* my patients, not because they blur boundaries but because they don't. They are the ones constantly telling us about this place—about their conversion disorder. They remind us that the unconscious does not speak with blurry lines but with absolute precision, with bodily force. We are the ones with the difficulty—giving ourselves over too much or too little in the struggle to listen.

Think about the stories I've just told you. Each one stops at a point. Each one has already within it the point at which to stop, usually at a place where meaning wears down—when history is so much, so excessive, that there isn't anything really to say. A point of chance rears its head, like a destiny, past, present, and future marked as a vanishing point on their body. Eye. Sour. Dim. Professional. Fragrant. Every patient I've spoken of—no matter how dramatic—hovers around this enigmatic point X, finding this place that is instinctually beyond operatics and soapboxes. The lure of drama is not the problem. Instead, we need to hear what lures them, what insists in their words, manifests in their body and through their symptoms in the transference. Here, laughter, absurdity, gesture, gathers the fibers of desire. This movement—like the hysteric throughout history—is the point of identification that defies identification. It forges an identification that manages somehow to efface itself almost immediately, opening onto the body. It is here that we find a means of separation. Only then to disappear.

VI

HYSTERICAL RUINOLOGY

Life, says someone somewhere, who is not an analyst, Étienne Gilson, is an unbroken power of active separations. I think after today's talk you won't confuse this remark with the one that is usually made with regard to frustrations. This is something quite different. This is about the limit point at which the place of lack is established.

—JACQUES LACAN, *ANXIETY*

HYSTERICAL RUINOLOGY

Can we take conversion out of the consulting room? Is the term, starting from the conundrum of sexuality and civilization, one we can use to understand something about our current moment? There is (thank god) already a philosopher who has done just this, reading the term "conversion" into a genealogy of history, especially the history of theology. What he discovers is that the body is not only the prime mover but *the* site of conflict as the place for the contestation of power. Giorgio Agamben also anticipates a psychoanalytic sense of history that is able to shift from a focus on the past to a focus on the present. His political theology allows for a thinking of conversion that pays close attention to more historical meanings, with a view toward aspects of a current crisis in the world, something Agamben pinpoints with the term "biopolitics," following Foucault.

The body moves front and center as the site of something original, concealed, and plastic, organizing power in the contemporary world, which is at odds with this something original—namely life, *bios*. Power, for Agamben, reaches further and further into our lives—it is aimed at our bodies, regulating them from the inside out, defining what counts as life and what does not. Now, power is disseminated on an invisible, cellular level. Agamben's intricate use of theological texts brings to the surface the sense of conversion as tied to religious transformation and the attempt to transform our ways of thinking about the world. He stretches conversion between its place in the history of religion and the permutations of today's biopolitical regime.

Psychoanalysis makes its appearance at strange points in Agamben's oeuvre, though it is never a conspicuous presence. The psychoanalytic conception of trauma for Agamben is linked to his way of conceiving crisis. Trauma, removed from its moment of terror, reappears as the inability to distinguish what is terrifying from what is not, calling forth all kinds of political machinations in the name of trying to draw this dividing line.[1] This is what is bad and this is what is good, this is what is me and this is what is not-me, this is a source of terror and this is not. Agamben's work zeroes in on the political sovereign, who is positioned beyond the law in a state of exception (2005), as the one who establishes or decides when the law is in effect or suspended. I read this as a question concerning the superego. Although the sovereign figure is in charge of containing terror, the sovereign itself becomes a terrifying figure given its exceptional position—the sovereign is a libido-fueled superego whose demand for regulation, sanitation, safety, and moral order overturns all order. For Agamben, this organization prevents the future from happening and is in fact aimed at maintaining the status quo by whatever means necessary. This is a post-traumatic defensive posture.

Following this, biopolitics is a perversion of religious conversion, which was originally a personal religious transformation. We begin to see how the religious sense of conversion should not be separated from some supposedly secular idea of transformation. The history of religion shows how theologians have rendered a particular temporality intrinsic to notions of salvation, redemption, and atonement. This way of thinking still exerts its influence in the present, in political and communal forms. Conversion could be read here as a subversion of the superego that brings the body back to life, that resurrects this body and returns it to some form of paradise.

In a more recent work, *The Signature of All Things* (2009), a collection of short essays on method, Agamben reminds his readers that any reflection on methodology cannot be done by the author, only by others, perhaps even only posthumously. Situating a methodology follows thought rather than precedes it, meaning that we write, think, and study in the dark without directive. This is to be contrasted with the outlines of so-called positive scientific research. This work on methodology—what he calls the study of paradigms and signatures and origins—must attempt to locate something behind, as it were, without knowing how to get there or what tools will be necessary. Agamben privileges the capacity simply for elaboration, for forms of interpretation that do not separate themselves from their current context or from their object of investigation: "It must retrace its own trajectory back to the point where something remains obscure and unthematized. Only a thought that does not conceal its own unsaid—but constantly takes it up and elaborates it—may eventually lay claim to originality" (8).

Agamben desires vigilance not over method but over the unsaid—what has remained hidden and unthematized. To do this, the work must move from singularity to singularity, case to case, transforming each of these into an example of a general rule that can never be stated a priori. This has deep echoes in a perhaps unspoken methodology of Freud, whose attention to the unconscious as something that can never be known directly gave him over to the study of cases, dreams, mistakes, and historical forms in order to try to say something about how this "unconscious" was structured.

The present is ordered in relation to a deep fracture, fault, or caesura. Every paradigm shift has the exemplary structure of revealing this fault anew. Agamben's major trilogy hones in on three singular cases that point to critical junctures in the history of politics, economics, communal life, and the law. Since hidden fractures organize the field of life, we must try to get as close to them as possible in order to see how they determine the movement of discourse across the centuries. In his first work of the trilogy, *Homo Sacer: Sovereign Power and Bare Life* (1995), the outlaw is a figure in politics, from Rome to the present, whose claim to sovereignty is always the extralegal power to decide on life and death, producing life as biopolitical life under the sway of the law. In tracing the outlaw, Agamben moves through Rome, the Holocaust, and contemporary politics.

In his second work, *The Kingdom and the Glory* (2011), the biopolitical points to an economy or economic libidinal order, close to what Agamben wants to call "life." The political relies on an economic field. One can see this more clearly when looking at religion, which overtly theorized the organization of power in relation to God around what was named "glory." These religious structures can be seen in the organization of government from bureaucracy and spectacle to media and ceremony. The distribution of power attempts to organize a fundamentally anarchic economy immanent to life—to contain, harness, or neutralize it, in a variety of theological forms.

The religious vision of redemption, according to Agamben, is our relief from biopolitical hierarchy and the stratification of life. Power finally rendered inoperative means that life can return to life. The final work of the trilogy, *The Highest Poverty: Monastic Rules and Form-of-Life* (2013), is centered on the history of monasticism and religious experiments in communal living as a foreshadowing of redemption. He sees in monasticism the attempt to find a form of life or living together that can render life autonomous and available for common use. Ethical life resists a system of law that tends to appropriate life, granting it to some and not others.

Every one of these changes or shifts in economy in the field of history has a quality of conversion insofar as it is an attempt to move a quantum of energy from one sphere of life to another, across this gap or fault. This movement is an attempt to try to make life equal to the forces of power, government, law, or community, which are the sedimentations of historical conversions. Conversion is increasingly counterproductive when the end becomes a further splitting or stratification of power rather than redemption. If there is an ideal in Agamben, it is messianic in structure, meaning not histories of the perfection of this or that structure but the end of history, the end of crisis.

The ideal would be imagining this potential opening as both a qualitative and quantitative change in a system that tends to avoid its own end. The system perpetuates splitting as a means of containment and avoidance. Conversion, in Agamben, is finally the victory of life against what he calls "bare life"[2] or contemporary nihilism and the destruction of experience. Agamben's notion of a coming community or a coming politics is thus an affirmation of life, of the world as it is, as irreparable, and, still, the ability to work without end. Life is reimagined as a disorder of conversion, the always incomplete conversions, with the goal of conversion nonetheless. In this way, I read Agamben's work as a history of conversion and his methodology as a hysterical archaeology, what I would like to call hysterical ruinology.

In his essay "Philosophical Archaeology" (2009), Agamben notes that the term "archaeology" first came from Kant. When considering the possibility of a philosophical history of philosophy—a philosophical archaeology—Kant ends up in the strange contradiction that it would have to be a study of the history of the thing that has not happened, since philosophy not only concerns itself with what is or has been but also what ought to or could have been. Philosophers, Kant says, build their work on the ruins of others, so any archeology of philosophy would be a "science of ruins," a ruinology whose object "can never truly be given as an empirical whole" (Agamben 2009, 82). The *archai* are what "could or ought to have been given and perhaps one day might be; for the moment, though, they exist only in the condition of partial objects or ruins" (82). With some impropriety, Agamben links this ruinology of Kant to Foucault's 1977 essay "Nietzsche, Genealogy, History," where Foucault's concept of genealogy is pitted against the search for origins, insofar as origins bring with them a "metahistorical deployment" and an "indefinite teleology" or, in other words, ideals, identity, and immobile forms seen not as partial objects or ruins but as original and determinate.

For Agamben, archaeology is a critique of tradition insofar as that tradition bars access to the sources that inform it:

> Provisionally, we may call "archaeology" that practice which in any historical investigation has to do not with the origins but with the moment of a phenomenon's arising and must therefore engage anew the sources and tradition. It cannot confront tradition without deconstructing the paradigms, techniques, and practices through which tradition regulates the forms of transmission, conditions access to sources, and in the final analysis determines the very status of the knowing subject.
>
> (89)

What kind of history, then, is archaeology or ruinology? Again, Agamben shifts the emphasis from the past—since there is no chronology or atemporal metahistory—toward what he calls the moment of arising, a point of disclosure that opens the present as what ought to or might have happened and so potentially still could. Asking us to abandon the goal of history or origins, we are to reach ever further toward the originary moment of splitting: "the revelation of the present as something that we were not able to live or think" (99). Agamben's strange combination of historical archaeology, philology, and philosophical theory deconstructs the status of the knowing subject.

Agamben reminds us that this eclipsing of the present follows Freud's concept of trauma and repression, in which an experience enters into a state of latency, where it is almost as if it hasn't happened or hasn't been experienced yet still insists in the present. But this is not a model of digging up original trauma. For Agamben, we have to find what is nonlived in a life, which he says happens at the limit between the past, the present, and the future—or at their point of indifference. Work is not a digging up of the past, as in the standard idea of archeology, but a hysterical ruinology where the future is buried in the past, in the mode of Heidegger's ecstatic temporality. What we have not lived overdetermines our life. Archeological work is not the establishment of facts—knowledge—but an act of clearing. The ruin opens the future: *Saxa loquuutur!* "The analogy between archeological regression and psychoanalysis now seems clearer" (102).

Is this not at the heart of what I am calling the psychoanalytic moment of conversion? Making stones speak their music of the future? It is with this understanding of history that Agamben returns to theological terminology such as redemption and salvation—to which I will add conversion—as not only aspects of religious discourse but as methods. What is of importance in the resurrection of these categories is the sense of the end of history, where the past to be salvaged is the inoperative past and where the act of salvation allows what is inoperative to finally speak:

> Contemporary politics is this devastating *experimentum linguae* that all over the planet unhinges and empties tradition and beliefs, ideologies and religions, identities and communities. Only those who succeed in carrying it to completion—without allowing what reveals to remain veiled in the nothingness that reveals, but bringing language itself to language—will be the first citizens of a community with neither presuppositions nor a State.
>
> (1993, 82.3)

Language, after its devastating failure to adhere to any lasting belief, finally is seen for what it is: unable to reveal anything but finding itself equal to itself. Language is not the unending game of concealment and half-revelations bound to an epistemology that chases eternity. Language is closer to what Agamben calls signature, name, singularity, and the destruction of spectacle. Those who take language for what it is will find another way to form a community.

AN ECONOMY OF SONG

In Agamben's *The Kingdom and the Glory* (2011), a general economy lies behind all conceptions of government, showing that there is no absolute substance of power, only a series of tensions or forces that are regulated and distributed, linking economy with the theological concept of glory. Providence is the name of the machine that attempts to unite the split halves in the *gubernatio dei*, the divine government of the world. God faces a corrupted and extraneous nature that needs to be redeemed. God is the name for the economy that has become inoperative when the world was split in two, something that we find symbolically in the image of the empty throne. Agamben finds in this image one of the most powerful, perhaps parodic, symbols for sovereign power: the king is dead, long live the king.

Moving from politics to theology to economy, Agamben demonstrates the successive attempts to conceal and contain this anarchic excess that he calls glory. If we make an unequivocal leap to psychoanalysis, the economic is the both origin and end for most psychoanalytic thought contained in Freud's theory of libido or the drive. Symptoms begin and end in Freud as a testament to an economic overhaul—they are reminders or remainders of blows to the psychical system that throw it into imbalance. Interestingly, the economic model of the mind is often thought of as a fallacy of the early Freud—the Freud of physiology and biological reductionism, the original Freud of "Project for a Scientific Psychology" ([1895] 1995).

The economic model is seen as totalizing and unable to resist a trend toward quantification and abstraction. More than this, it is a mythological language of energy, a mechanistic idea of pain, pleasure, tension, and discharge. Nevertheless, the economic model in Freud is essentially the attempt at a science of libido and is not simply negligible. It embodies the project of psychoanalysis—in particular, as a project that resists displacements away from this hard, biosexual, and bodily theoretical core. "Happiness," as Freud wrote in *Civilization and Its Discontents*, "in the reduced sense in which we recognize it as possible, is a problem of the economics of the individual's libido" ([1930] 1995, 83).

Psychoanalysis is about movement, circulation, opening, including work with its negative underside: stasis, repression, resistance, repetition, defense, and closure. Clinical work tells us something about how the transfer from one to the other becomes possible for a patient in the work of analysis. Illness in Freud is even at times thought of as a displacement or shift from the quantitative to the qualitative or, in other words, the neurotic move from economy to meaning, from libido to defense. Change might be seen as a return or re-return to the economic or quantitative dimension of life, what many Lacanians underscore with their emphasis on *jouissance*.

Are we not always already talking about change with respect to changes in the pathways of libido? Why have we divorced qualitative change from one of quantity? Can we sustain a word like "sublimation," the idea of a displacement of sexuality with the full quantum of sexual satisfaction, without thinking economically? What happens to the drive when it is shorn of this economic dimension? Do we enter into a phantasmagoric structure whenever we ignore the economic? Is this the shift enacted by the symptom par excellence? These questions underscore the importance of thinking through the question of the economic.

To say it like this can sound too simple, but it is the simplicity that intrigues me. In a way, the economic is a means of cutting through the machinations of meaning or the enmeshment of interpretation and fantasy. Economically speaking, there is a crisis with respect to one's libido—an incomplete overhaul—seen when a patient is caught in a repetition. The repetition is looking for a way to complete the original crisis. Psychoanalytic work finds a way to cut this repetition, opening a new pathway on the level of the drive. In fact, this cut exposes the drive, exposes both patient and analyst to its sheer economic dimension. This happens not by virtue of meaning but in spite of it. All Lacanian knotting and unknotting takes its resonance here.

The tact of the analyst runs counter to the futile game of a causal system of meaning, the deployment of metahistorical realities, and instead we learn how to handle or bear the tension generated within the analytic process. What closes down possibility faster than one could say the word is usually the analyst's own resistances to the pressures of the analytic situation—in particular, the pressure that builds because of transference. The best means for relieving this tension: discharge and displacement via more meaning!

This economic language is best exemplified in Freud by the language of tension. It contains, says Philip Rieff, the great American sociological interpreter of Freud, "a moral judgment far more powerful than any quantitative index the terms might suggest. . . . [It] compose[s] a vast ethical metaphor" (1959, 130). This follows, as Rieff points out, much of Nietzsche's thought on the question of value. In *The Will to Power* (1901), Nietzsche states that value is only a standpoint insofar as it describes a multiplicity of forces, their increase and diminution a veritable becoming, which it only impotently expresses. If the economic isn't a problem, it might be a virtue.

If there is a reason to return to the economic model, it is in light of this virtue of unrelentingly describing everything on the basis of heterogeneous forces that leave us—our knowledge, our morality, and our political agendas—out of it. There isn't any knowledge at this point. The analyst is a temporary container of libido, its cause of overflow. The analyst is a body caught in transference. We need not determine the transference otherwise. To grasp what provokes desire through the sheer movements of quantity that it implies is enough. To add anything more would begin to obstruct possibility, which is to say that to recognize the economic is to recognize the ethical limit that it underscores in relation to epistemology.

It is with the economic factor of mental life that Freud puts any hope in the future, namely, the ways in which an individual and society might accommodate the heterogeneity of economic drive life, the specificity of being a body with history. It is this singular dimension that Freud underscores as being distinctly different from the eternal struggle of life and death, which most social-psychoanalytic theorists place at the center of conflict within civilization. Rather, one might see instead that what we resist is this specific materiality of the economic as the ground of the unconscious, as the place where we get our hands dirty in the day-to-day work as a psychoanalyst. We do not, Freud cautions, do anything for the grand struggle of life versus death.

One can find this conundrum in Agamben's investigation into the figure of the angel, which is the representative of economy or economic life. Angels are representatives of what cannot be represented, they are the face, body, or voice God reveals to man of an economy foreign to human systems of representation and meaning. Their activity is depicted as song, hymn, liturgy, praise, and glory, often prophetic or oracular: uniting speech and action, announcing another order of time, and playing an important role in the second coming or the reconciliation of God with the world. Angels announce the coming community.

In a later theological rendering, these angelic figures become part of a system of government and bureaucracy, making angels mediators or legislators or bureaucrats, stationed between the divine and human kingdom. The angelic *ministirium* covers the original angelic *mysterium*; Agamben is interested in this historical shift from mystical tradition to a bureaucratic one. Aquinas, Agamben says, asked the question: What happens to angels once their duty has been fulfilled? What happens to angels after the Day of Judgment? For some, the angels disappear: "With every providential operation exhausted and with all administration of salvation coming to an end, only song remains" (2011, 162). We enter into the pure life of economy. There is no chasm to cross any longer, and government is rendered inoperative.

Agamben writes of this cessation: "Glory occupies the place of postjudicial inoperativity; it is the eternal amen in which all works and all divine and human words are resolved" (239). "Amen" means both "enough" and "yes." Glory is this fascinating remainder when work as defense can be brought to an end. Doxa will leave the sphere of opinion and return to the kingdom as glory. In my reading of Agamben's angels, they are both the hysteric and the hysterical symptom, a figure that represents the points of crisis in the economic dimension or the relation between God and humanity. Conversion disorder speaks to what is impossible at this intersection of history and eternity, the angels singing (or perhaps laughing) a forgotten anarchic autonomy of life against law.

THE ANALYST IS PULLING OUT

In the fight between life and law, Jesus is the figure of reconciliation and another urgent point of investigation. Agamben focuses on the trial of Jesus as a crossing between "the temporal and the eternal, and between the divine and the human, [which] assumed precisely the form of a *krisis*, that is, of a juridical trial," a trial that continues within every contemporary crisis (2015, 2). In a close analysis of the text and an investigation into centuries of contradictory scholarship, Agamben hones in on one thing: that neither Pilate, a judge legally invested with earthly power, nor Jesus, made a judge through scorn, representing another kingdom and another world, truly pronounce a judgment: "The radical critique of every judgment is an essential part of Jesus's teaching: 'Do not judge (*me krinete*), so that you may not be judged' (Matthew 7:1) . . . the eternal does not want to judge the world but to save it; at least until the end of time judgment and salvation mutually exclude one another" (38). Why must the one who will not judge be subjected to the judgment of an earthly judge? What is this mysterious and carefully articulated drama between Pilate and Jesus?

Pilate and Jesus, for Agamben, represent the antithesis or caesura between economy and history, temporality and eternity, justice and salvation. They are this contradiction. Theology in the fifth and sixth centuries struggled to reconcile and legitimate church and king, whose unity is betrayed by the thesis of the king's two bodies or two wills—earthly and divine. That two-part thesis is allegorically preceded by the critical encounter of Jesus with Pilate (Kantorowicz 1957). The doctrine of two wills, Agamben points out, is hypocritical, since you can always use one to justify the other. But does this follow from the legal drama between Jesus and Pilate? What we find in the encounter is the irreconcilable itself: neither Jesus nor Pilate can pronounce a judgment. Pilate remains resolutely undecided:

> They end up in a common, indecisive, and undecidable, *non liquet*. To testify, here and now, to the truth of a kingdom that is not here means accepting that what we want to save will judge us. This is because the world in its fallenness, does not want salvation but justice. And it wants it precisely because it is not asking to be saved. As unsavable, creatures judge the eternal: this is the paradox that in the end, before Pilate, cuts Jesus short. Here is the cross; here is history.
>
> (Agamben 2015, 45)

This little exegesis on Pilate and Jesus demonstrates that the human being is condemned to an incessant *krisis*, a trial without resolution, because nothing can be decided once and for all.

What is of greatest importance cannot be judged or saved; it remains obscure. This radical incommensurability between juridical and divine registers forms the backdrop to a world that unites these divided figures in governmental power—especially the absolute power over life and death. Power is the attempt at an absolute decision or judgment that is also supposed to leave decisions about life and death to God. Think of the current state of government—incessant decisions on nothing, or at least on nothing of any real consequence, yet with decisions about life and death always in the background.

What, you might ask, has any of this to do with psychoanalysis? What fascinated me is that the absolute figure of religious conversion, Jesus, becomes not a conversion into a decisive day of reckoning, not the arrival of a certain moral order, nor even a figure of salvation, but the absence of all these: the revelation of the irreparable, the undecidable, poverty, constant *krisis*, disorder, and division. Agamben likens this to the psychoanalytic notion of trauma: separated from its original moment, forced into latency, it becomes a permanent condition. Judgment, in deciding on the undecidable, reverses what is properly nothing into a potential catastrophe. Jesus—whose decision is grounded in another world—decides on nothing and does not judge.

It is in light of this reading that I want to bring forward a question regarding the function of the analyst. In Lacan's late, nearly impossible-to-read essay "L'étourdit" (1972a), the *dire*, *dit*, or saying is emphasized against what is said and what is heard. Lacan is looking for the voice, the real voice, before it is sedimented into a "said." The famous line reads: the saying remains forgotten behind what is said in what is heard. While this formula might read as an assertion, it is in fact modal or existential, something that a patient attests to. In other words, it itself is an act of saying and speaks to what an analyst must listen to, not what should be said about analysis, taking the form of a law. How can psychoanalysis keep the voice alive, keep the voice from reifying into something that establishes what has supposedly been said? What role does the other play when transforming the saying into something said? Psychoanalysis, the impossible profession, is centered on this act of saying. What does it do but speak in a way that is meant to have consequences?

Patients constantly speak to their disappointment with interpretations—even when good—as if something has closed down that had only a moment before opened. They speak about how upon hearing an interpretation they veer away almost immediately from a moment in which they really found themselves speaking. Saying has to carry, in some way, its own disappearance, including disappointment with this diminishing rate of return. This late essay of Lacan's has been likened to Joyce in the attempt to keep the act of saying—the quality of voice, the noise, its grain—more alive than any set of meanings. This saying, Lacan goes on, is what can bring us face to face with the impossible, which is the goal of psychoanalysis.

Meaning, that what can be said as said, will never face a limit. Meaning cannot encounter what is impossible within its own structure:

> If I had recourse this year to the first, namely, to set theory, it was to refer to it the marvelous efflorescence which by isolating the incomplete from the inconsistent in logic, the indemonstrable from the refutable,

and even adding to it the undecidable, by not managing to exclude itself from demonstrability, puts us face to face with the impossible so that there could be ejected the "that's not it" which is the wail of an appeal to the real.

(Lacan 1972a, 40)

The incomplete, the inconsistent, and the undecidable—something Lacan also likens to scraps of words, the lability of language, and something he names "joy" (from Freud to Joyce in "L'étourdit")—are what psychoanalysis brings to the surface in searching for this "saying." These carry the impossible with them and strike out against any sedimentation of knowledge, including the notion of a final judgment, which requires a presupposition.

In this essay, Lacan intertwines mathematical logic with the qualities of speaking with a purity of voice that can appear in an analytic session. It is one of the rare times that Lacan forces his topological logic to work directly on the clinical encounter, rather than leaving these as one iteration among others. Lacan, in an aside, distinguishes the impossible in saying from what he calls "the wail of an appeal to the real" (1972a, 40). He seems fed up with the fascination of the hysteric with the impossible, heard in her ever-present complaint "that's not it." We are at the point of a final showdown between the hysteric and the analyst—what Freud called its bedrock.

The torsion of the analyst away from the hysteric's abject complaint is important in this essay because, for Lacan, her abjection is implicated in the failures of the psychoanalytic institution, including the failure to retain the saying of Freud. The hysteric, Lacan seems to say, simply pronounces a "that's not it." Akin to hysterical disgust with the sexual nature of any act, she uses her power of negation not to say anything herself except that this isn't what she wants. Even if this is a fortunate crossroads where the analyst is able to ask the patient "what do you want?", without this intervention her nothing solidifies into a monolithic said as problematic as codifying Freud's work.

Lacan says that it is from the saying of Freud that every analyst must take their formation—their point of conversion. The saying of Freud is not what Freud said. The analyst could be saved from the force of reification because discourse will always reject them—this is what he means by the incomplete, the inconsistent, and the undecidable. To reduce Freud to what he said or, in the case of our hysteric, what Freud didn't say, is somehow to bypass this rejection. Through the desire for inclusion, on the one hand, being the one to say what was heard in his saying, or counter-rejection, on the other, being the one to say what should have been said by virtue of what was not, Lacan differentiates the position of the analyst.

We do not set up another collective mythology, even if it is the bond of the abject. We speak to one another. In a touching moment, Lacan declares that every analyst can maintain a tie to Freud's saying, something he says "would have held them," as opposed to the other discourses in which this saying is rejected or barred (1972a, 44). Freud's act of saying is tied to the extraordinary transgression implied in the discovery of the unconscious, of announcing this *non liquet*. Freud discovers something that will always reject him, something that will always exceed him. Freud discovers something that amounts to nothing. Freud founds a work that cannot function as a system easily transmitted between generations yet is about the essence of transmission.

What the psychoanalyst transmits, and how, must be reinvented again and again. We can perhaps see this ethos most clearly when Lacan reestablishes Freud's saying in his Irma dream:

> I am he who wants to be forgiven for having dared to begin to cure these patients, who until now no one wanted to understand and whose cure was forbidden . . . I am he who wants not to be guilty of it for to transgress any limit imposed up to now on human activity is always to be guilty. I want not to be born that . . . Here I am only the representative of this vague, vast movement, the quest for truth, in which I efface myself. I am no longer anything. My ambition was greater than I . . . and precisely to the extent that I desired it too much, that I partook in this action, that I wanted to be, myself, the creator, I am not the creator. The creator is someone greater than I. It is my unconscious, it is this voice which speaks in me, beyond me.
>
> (1991, 170–171)

This is the moment that establishes the transference to Freud as a transference to psychoanalysis: a potential bond between analysts to continue the project of psychoanalysis. We psychoanalysts are the castoffs of language, yet we need to distance ourselves from the promise of rejection that being an analyst offers, much like we distance ourselves from the surprising access we are granted to love. This is the other side of the continued work offered by a transference to psychoanalysis.

Our susceptibility to rejection from our very own medium (saying) can take the form of rejecting this rejection or wallowing in it. The vicissitudes of the latter, some kind of psychoanalytic hysterical whining, are the most dangerous. Those who reject psychoanalysis, in the end, simply leave. But for those who stay bound to a complaint or lament, this will have irrevocable effects on the field:

> What I denounce, is that everything is used by analysts of this stock to file off from a challenge that I hold they take their existence from—for there is a fact of structure that determines them. The challenge I denote as abjection. We know that the term absolute has haunted knowledge and power—derisorily we have to say: there it seemed, remained the hope that the saints represent elsewhere. We must become disenchanted by it. The analyst is pulling out.
>
> (1972b, 23–24)

The challenge is the challenge of abjection, a pathos that haunts all knowledge and power. This is something categorically excluded from the position of the analyst for Lacan. So much so that the abject position of the saint is also denounced by Lacan as one more absolute.[3]

The caricature of the "melancholic analyst" who, after so many years of schooling and so many years of practice, feels depressed by the repetitive nature of clinical conundrums, is being addressed by Lacan here. You have Jesus who has been forsaken by his father and masochistically turns the other cheek, and you have Jesus who is steadfast in his refusal to judge. The choice between the father-pathos of masochism and the inability to judge haunts the impossible professions, namely, those professions that rely on transference and speech and not power or, by extension, knowledge. Given that for Lacan the abject haunts all knowledge and power, and given that the discourse of the analyst is an attempt to separate oneself from this, all analysts must pass through this challenge of abjection or melancholia. From this challenge, the analyst must pull out. "I am neither consoled nor desolated by it," Lacan says of the analytic institution (1972b, 23).

Insofar as we know that our voice, our act of saying produces effects, we can remain psychoanalysts. Simply that. To speak from the position of saying is the only position that has the possibility of a real effect—not knowledge, not power. The effect of the analyst's voice should be contrasted with the effects of the superego—surely they are all on the same, very fine line, but perhaps the crucial point is the separation between speech and knowledge or mere power. Yes, saying is an act, an act that surely affects us deeply, sometimes even with great terror—the voice of our parents like angry gods—yet it is up to the analyst to find the way to bring the superego from terror to speech. Superegoic rejection, the threats levied by each one of us, ultimately aren't personal, Lacan claims. They are simply using the point of rejection inside speech itself, to which we are all subjected.

Lacan plays with three figures of the impossible: judgment, the sexual relationship, and sense. Judgment feels the most crucial, not only given our historical moment but also in terms of what it means to be an analyst in relation to the troubled psychoanalytic institution. The superego attacks at the place where body and word are finally indistinguishable—at the point of the life of a saying. The voice is the final object in Lacan's series—oral, anal, phallic, gaze, voice—and it is certainly the most obscure in the psychoanalytic literature. It always seems to arise at the final moments of analysis, this question of what has been heard or said, rearing its head at the place where some ambiguity in this exchange cannot be dispensed with.

In the unraveling of fantasy, it is within the kernel of speech that judgment is held in place. Agamben has shown that the oath (a verbal saying between parties) is the original form of the law. Judgment unravels not by establishing itself securely in an oath that holds as a written law but rather by touching something real on the level of voice, and like a breaking point or moment of conversion, judgment loses all meaning.

"Insult, since it proves through the epos to be the first as well as the last word of dialogue, judgment, likewise, up to the 'Last,' remains a phantasy, and to say it, only touches on the real by losing all meaning" (1972b, 17). It is simply two people speaking. It was always two people only speaking, like Jesus and Pilate. The analyst, Lacan says, must know how to make himself a conduit of this transformation where the power of judgment within a patient's neurotic guilt suddenly loses all meaning, crumbles, and drops.

Lacan's focus on this encounter with what is impossible can also be read alongside Freud's picture of the child's sexual research. Freud says that the child cannot understand the vaginal orifice, the role of intercourse, or the inseminating role of semen. Silly and perhaps a bit crude, but isn't this the truth of sexual research? Aren't these childish questions directed at the place on the body that marks women and sense, love and sexual relationships, and judgment and authority? The superego—the force of judgment or salvation—is nothing other than the attempt at levying a response to these three impossible points around which so much morality has been attached, attempting to find an anchor in our flesh. From this, Lacan says, the analyst must pull out. An apt and rather sardonic metaphor, if it even is a metaphor.

When patients tell you about this fabric of the impossible that overlies their lives, no meaning can be added, no salvific narrative, even when the demand is directed more and more toward the analyst. One of my patients upped the ante precisely at this point; it concerned a question of my voice and her desire for a judgment. She wanted me to confirm for her that her mother had abused her, something that she was told by a friend who was a psychic. The question of belief, belief in what she is saying, belief in her pain and what has happened to her, and indeed, spiritual belief was, from the beginning of this analysis, a condensed hinge in the transference. People hadn't believed her, it is true.

In session, she would watch my face carefully for the signs of what she took to be belief. I was waiting for this subtle game to erupt in crisis. After a series of angry episodes in which she increasingly tried to lock me down, to pinpoint inconsistencies in what she heard in what I said, accompanied by fits of violent screaming and attempts to end the treatment, something broke. "Why do you need me to join you here? Why can I not continue to listen, to continue to try to speak with you, without an absolute affirmation that I don't believe is mine to give? Because I believe you, not because I don't!" She stopped screaming. "Because I would be so alone in this." Indeed, she is.

Let me end with a particularly moving dream by a patient. She is handed two pills by a powerful and successful business woman. One pill will impregnate her with this woman's child—her body is spent, and she needs a host. The other pill is part of a trial, and there is no certainty as to whether it will have any effect at all. While there is much to say about the dream and its place in this woman's analysis, what is important for us here is the fascinating way the dream underlines the two meanings inherent in the word "trial"—trial as the procedure for establishing certainty or judgment and trial as test with an uncertain outcome, trying something on without a guarantee.

There is something very Agambenian about her premonition that the trial as judgment is this takeover of her body, using the other's life for one's own end to make up for what has been spent on the wider system. There is, she acknowledged, a comfort in the guaranteed ends. She will be pregnant, even if that is at her own expense. This is contrasted with a position where no judgment is possible, where the means must be followed without end, where she has only what she tries. The force of a longstanding violent melancholia lay with the former, whereas her cure in the analysis, I believe, was pointing her toward the latter possibility.

VII

COITUS INTERRUPTUS

Hence the necessity of converting reflexive language. It must be directed not toward any inner confirmation—not toward a kind of central, unshakable certitude—but toward an outer bound where it must continually contest itself. When language arrives at its own edge, what it finds is not a positivity that contradicts it, but the void that will efface it. Into that void it must go, consenting to come undone in the rumbling, in the immediate negation of what it says, in a silence that is not the intimacy of a secret but a pure outside where words endlessly unravel.

—MICHEL FOUCAULT, *THE THOUGHT FROM OUTSIDE*

COITUS INTERRUPTUS

Of all the silly psychoanalytic ideas laid bare for the world to see, perhaps none is as easily derided as the notion that anxiety is a result of *coitus interruptus*—a terrible cliché, alongside Freud's other early childish theories of sexuality, like the ones involving menstrual cycles and the nose. When it comes to anxiety in particular, Freud seems to need the link between neurotic angst and the hard body of biology—some grain of the drive there to give substance to what is purely psychological, existential, and thus nebulous in the phenomenon of anxiety.

Yet anxiety for Freud is a foolproof argument against any easy Darwinian perspective because it embodies evolution gone haywire, the involuting effects of the civilizing function of society, and, simply, the sheer problem of sex. Anxiety alerts us to neurosis better than even the hysteric can, for, at the very least, anxiety is something everyone knows about. Solutions are whispered about along backchannels: methods of preventing conception and the delirious fear of an explosion of something unwanted—not on the inside but always on the outside.

Anxiety, like neurasthenia or the taboo on virginity, is linked to the failure of the sexual and grounds the demand for conversion. Orgasm, Freud tells us, is the ejection into the outside of scraps or grains of libido, the exteriorization of the drive in bodily coitus. Anxiety is these scraps trapped on the inside, unable to enter the stream of thought or simply to return to the body, caught between here and nowhere. One can begin to see why *coitus interruptus* was an intriguing proposition—an image of the incomplete act, leaving something cut off midstream. Anxiety, both body and not body at once or, perhaps better, inhabiting the thin line between the two, speaks to some impossible process taking place between a body and the world, my body and yours.

The theory of anxiety is an unwitting nod to the intersubjective matrix of the mind.[1] While Freud is developing the earliest threads of his theory of the pleasure principle, the question of anxiety and orgasm hovers in the background, tied to a deep desire in Freud for etiological explanations—like *coitus interruptus*—that are also diagnoses of culture. The structure of the drive must also be a question of social and historical configurations. The whole sexual apparatus of anxiety in Freud is not merely anxiety about sex or because of sex, though that comes up, but instead confirms the tight relationship between sexuality and anxiety in the determination of social forms. What do we do with anxiety?

Freud makes anxiety a half-enjoyed interruption, the stoppage of orgasm, the strange choice of this anxious pain against the pain of uninterrupted or complete enjoyment—fulfillment with a degree of irony. Anxiety is the choice to reinternalize the drive against what Freud concretely sees as its most absolute form of externalization, namely, orgasm or pregnancy. If we neither easily submit to nor reject what is so outright silly about this notion of externalization, what we can see are the lineaments of Freud's later theory of sublimation in this necessity for anxiety to exteriorize itself in some manner.

To some extent, the choice is between a perverse relationship to anxiety and a neurotic one. Perversion triumphs insofar as it seeks to put anxiety out there, to act it out. The pervert has been characterized as the figure who externalizes anxiety by making it belong exclusively to the other person, by making *them* anxious about sex—unveiling their anxious desire while keeping their own at a remove. The neurotic, on the other hand, stands still, refusing to confront the outside, screening out any involvement with the other or making them an object of hate or repugnance. If the drive must be crystallized externally, what form might this take? What transformation of our own anxiety is possible? While Freud quickly moves away from the theory of *coitus interruptus*, he will wrestle with anxiety all his life.

Anxiety is not a question of delineating something absolutely on the inside—something that anxiety nevertheless promises, as if there is nothing more interior or original than anxiety. Rather, anxiety is about how to place something outside. In this original link between anxiety and *coitus interruptus*, Freud links anxiety to something external—this goes against the superficial conclusion that fear is about an external danger while anxiety concerns an internal one. What is inside, what is outside, what is in between the two, what parts of us are ours, and what belongs to whom are not easy to distinguish. Anxiety alerts us to these problems.

If we read Freud's correspondence with Fliess and his early musings on *coitus interruptus* and anxiety, he focuses on the alienation experienced between the somatic and the psychical, which is embodied by the choice of protection against conception or the hesitation around the repercussions of intercourse and the inability to find "adequate satisfaction in a secure relationship" (Freud 1985, 93). It's not clear what he means by this, especially "a secure relationship," but the point is that the patient seems to choose a half-pleasure rather than no pleasure or full pleasure. This half-choice erodes one's somatic sexual constitution over time, leading Freud into a tight symptomatic loop: anxiety erupts because of interrupted pleasure, and anxiety leads one to interrupt pleasure.

Masturbation becomes the hallmark of ruined libidinal potential; it leads to a weakened constitution, weakened potency, and eventually a disposition to anxiety, pessimism, and low self-confidence. Freud sometimes described this as actual neurosis, whose three subtypes were neurasthenia (libidinal depletion), anxiety neurosis, and hypochondria. Freud even reacts with surprise to a man who would choose *coitus interruptus* when he seems to desire his wife and at the time had only two children. This man, he writes, has "coitus every twelve to fourteen days or so; often, too, with long intervals. Admits that he feels limp and wretched after coitus with a condom; but not immediately afterwards, only two days later—or, as he puts it, he has noticed that two days later he gets digestive trouble. Why does he use a condom? One should not have too many children! ([He has] two)" (94). The repetition of the signifier "two" is remarkable, including coitus every two weeks, stomachaches two days later, and two children, but what Freud is attempting to understand, at least at this early point, is why the man uses a condom. He only has two children!

Freud is fixated on the practicality of the sexual practices and not how they are embedded in a set of signifiers. His conclusions in cases like this one are, oddly, invariably stacked against the men. Males, Freud claims, are more likely to develop these libidinal problems in the first decades of adult sexual life, women in the second (how ill-timed the sexes are). Why? In part because of masturbation, in part because of moral strictures, in part because of fear of infection and pregnancy. Only later will he take note of the hint of a problem in relation to one's desire, but it is there, and Freud points to it via his obsession with *coitus interruptus*.

Desire, so important to Freud's later theories, is hinted at in the case of a man, Herr K, who fell in love with a woman who "was a flirt, a great shock when he heard she was engaged to someone else. Now no longer in love—he attaches little importance to it—he went on" (90–91). After his first intercourse with her, he had an anxiety attack that night and a few days later. He uses a condom, often feels limp after. His libido has diminished over the last year. In yet another case, Freud described a similar situation: "The man's libido has been diminishing . . . the preparations for using a condom are enough to make him feel that the whole act is something forced on him and his enjoyment of it is something he was persuaded into. This is no doubt the nub of the whole business" (93). For both these men, sexual encounters early on with women caused an increase in somatic excitation, which could not be mastered, leading to an overall weakness in psychical mastery over somatic excitation, contributing to its more rapid degeneration in an already weakened system. The decision to use a condom for fear of infection comes after the fact—what Freud says laid the "foundation for what I have described as the factor of alienation between the somatic and psychical" (93).

The man, Freud says, "brought psychical sexual weakness on himself by spoiling coitus for himself" (93). Spoiling one's sexual life ultimately weakens the psychical and then the physical. At the end of the discussion, Freud is interested in the short attacks of melancholic mood, which he speculates must be of importance to his actual neurosis, which is caused by alienation—but "for the moment I can only make note of it" (93). What *is* important to note is how early all of this is: 1894. We are still six years away from the publication of *The Interpretation of Dreams*. Yet in this little case vignette we can see that far from being a description of actual neurosis, it seems like a rather typical case of obsessional melancholia, replete with all the problems of rectifying such patients' relation to desire.

These men choose to spoil coitus on every occasion or to feel forced and persuaded, as if it wasn't their own desire. This bears a relationship to a choice and a pleasure experienced in the past that went awry—especially for the one who had been cuckolded—marking and undoing that choice with every half-decision, or half-enjoyment, through *coitus interruptus*. This, for Freud, feels entirely masculine, and, in fact, he concludes on several occasion in his letters to Fliess that women seem to be less disposed to this version of neurasthenic actual neurosis—"normally girls are sound"—or they are only neurasthenic in the case of the inability to get pregnant, bad marriages with neurasthenic men, or approaching menopause.

One ought to be careful when considering a woman's complaints over anxiety, Freud cautions; more often than not they are married to neurasthenic men who are making them hysterical.[2] And the more passionate a woman, the more she will react to the decrease in a man's potency, the vicissitudes of *coitus interruptus*, and fall ill. He contrasts this form of neurasthenia in women, or in women with low libidos who could tolerate this situation more easily, to men's neurasthenia. Here we find a complete inversion between male and female reactions to *coitus interruptus*—passionless men cannot tolerate it, passionless women can, passionate women cannot, and passionate men can. Anxiety, Freud concludes, is in close relation with sexual limitation. The more impudent and daring, the more one is likely to indulge sexually and thereby fend off neurotic illness and the vicissitudes of inhibition in the form of hesitation, self-protection, dissatisfaction, and even the kind of pessimistic melancholic mood that comes with the blows to confidence that anxiety exacts.

Again, we are very close to his 1921 conclusion from *Group Psychology and the Analysis of the Ego* that sexual satisfaction is on the side of reality. In this early moment in Freud's reflections on anxiety, he levies a surprising indictment at culture: "In the absence of such a solution [innocuous methods of preventing conception and disease], society appears doomed to fall a victim to incurable neuroses, which reduce the enjoyment of life to a minimum, destroy the marriage relation and bring hereditary ruin on the whole coming generation" (1985, 44). *Coitus interruptus* is destroying the family, to say nothing of a whole generation to come, and even the lower strata—meaning the less civilized and so less neurotic—Freud says will succumb. Neurasthenia is the future of civilization, a world of hesitant half-orgasming men and more and more hysterical women. The end, or truth, of marriage is hereditary ruin.

If the beginning half of *Civilization and Its Discontents* is concerned with this intertwined relationship between pleasure and society, unpleasure and anxiety, the second half signals the changes wrought by Freud's second topology, which hones in on the problem of trauma, repetition, the superego, guilt, and aggression. But despite all his banging on about the death drive, Freud still sees a solution in the power of psychoanalysis to push back against the costs wrought by civilization against desire. Freud imagines the possibility of a civilization that could accommodate the *something unique* in one's libidinal economy. These solutions by psychoanalysis, or even new societal forms, are as equally on the outside as this original imagined solution of an innocuous method of preventing conception or disease, or what he comically prescribes as the easy and early access for young boys to good girls, making *coitus interruptus* unwarranted.

When looking at Freud's second topological model, he famously changes his theory of anxiety, making it the accomplice of the ego rather than of the libido and placing it before repression, not subsequent to it. Repression becomes the solution to anxiety. Freud divides anxiety into two moments: the first is a result of trauma, the ego being overwhelmed by stimuli it was unable to prepare for or defend against; the second is a response to trauma, trying to master it, to turn passivity into activity, by anticipating danger, sending out preparatory signals that take the form of anxiety. Fixation on the first moment is closer to actual neurosis, a system overwhelmed, while the second is psychoneurotic, a system based in backlash—though both end up using the strategy of avoidance. Small doses of anxiety are an attempt to preserve the status quo, to inoculate against further danger. Otherwise, the individual must turn away entirely from the overly exciting stimulus. In both cases, we can see that repression isn't operating well, which is why there is anxiety in the place where there ought to be the *belle indifference* of the symptom. The symptom is a metabolization of trauma—a representative or a strange form of memory. The symptom is a structure; anxiety is the devastation of the structure, which is what actual neurosis essentially signifies.

While this is certainly a twist in the tale of anxiety that Freud is telling, he does eventually say that these changes aren't really at odds with his original thesis. Libidinal tension makes the ego helpless, which is essentially how he defines trauma and the concomitant response of signal anxiety. In both the original and the second model, what is discharged as anxiety, he says, is *surplus* libido, and the economic implications are always the same— this surplus creates helplessness and anxiety. Rather than repression and the symptom folding outside and inside together, anxiety is the strange inside-out problem of overstimulation, avoidance, and helplessness. While this might be disconcerting because it might represent some degradation of the beautiful model of the mind in repression and symptom formation, something here deserves our attention.

Freud says that many have noted the relationship between anxiety and self-preservation, or anxiety and the fear of death, something that is certainly in the ego's wheelhouse. In these moments, he is fighting Rank's theory that anxiety comes from the trauma of birth, from the separation from the mother's body.[3] He is quick to dismiss Rank because, he says, "nothing resembling death can be experienced," and if it is simply birth trauma, then why wouldn't everyone be cripplingly anxious ([1926] 1995, 130)? What we are witnessing with anxiety is a psychosexual problem, not an existential one.

What the ego does know, Freud says, are the losses and separations that hinge on psychosexual development. In fact, this is where we see anxiety in childhood, the first being separation anxiety in the infant once the representation of the mother has cohered enough for the child to imagine losing her. This occurs well after any supposed birth trauma and is linked less to the expulsion from the uterine environment and more to the nature of a representational mind and the consequences of pleasure. "At birth," writes Freud, "no object existed and so no object could be missed" (203).

Repression mirrors the original condition of being without an object because the object—or object tie—is erased. With anxiety, on the other hand, the object tie is preserved but under the signal of apprehension concerning one's threatened attachment to it. The symptom is a return to objectlessness, or the symptom replaces the anxious tie to the object. The choice, oddly enough, seems to be between anxiety linked to an unwavering attachment to the object with no mind or an object loss that mirrors the original objectless disposition through a symptomatic construction that creates the container called mind.

In a moment I find rather surprising, Freud reverses cause and effect entirely, saying that anxiety is not about the expectation of a danger but the experience of and reaction to a specific loss or separation. This shifts the emphasis from the imagined danger to the nature of the tie to the object. Here, Freud evokes an affective chain that begins with anxiety and is followed by helplessness, pain, mourning, then separation. He then wonders how he could have arrived at this conclusion, since the reaction to loss and separation is pain and mourning, not anxiety. It is a question of undoing the ties that bind—what he calls decathexis. Separation is an achievement, one opposed to anxiety and related to the work of mourning, which allows one to decathect an attachment to a lost object.

It is here that we must return to the question of surplus libido discharged as anxiety. Whether one experiences curtailed enjoyment or the fear of libidinal satisfaction, whether the ego is overwhelmed by internal or external stimuli it cannot master, whether the system is going haywire and interpreting everything as a signal of danger or anticipating danger or fearing separation from a beloved, there is a surplus in relation to an object, and this surplus takes the form of anxiety, from which one must separate. Freud implies the necessity for working over or working through in the form of a substitute object through displacement and loss or in the form of a satisfaction reached in another mode of relating to an object. What is necessary either way is to reduce this excess of helplessness, which is equivalent to whatever Freud means by separation. We may even call this "common human unhappiness." This reduction, which carries the force of separation, must be created.

This tale of anxiety reveals something about the stakes of an analytic cure. Freud's attempt to clarify the nature of anxiety leads him to consider what is distinct about the human relationship to objects, especially insofar as this tie is always sexual. In one sense, we might link this to the question of conversion, since all modes of attachment to objects seem to be either pathologically anticipatory or retroactively symptomatic, and thus a new form of relation must be created. How can we live with less anxiety and more pleasure, or how do we convert one to the other?

For Lacan, anxiety emerges at the place where separation is a question. Freud was already beginning to allude to this at the end of *Inhibitions, Symptoms, and Anxiety* (1926). He draws out the impulse to decathect the object and the anxious reaction that can be provoked by this call. If Freud folds anxiety into a developmental table—fear of the loss of the object, fear of the loss of the object's love, castration anxiety, or superego threats—Lacan reads these steps as the anxieties of being an object for the other, certainly something the child experiences. We are taken by others as a body, taken in by their enjoyment, and we lend out parts of ourselves to others. Lacan transforms the question of the object into the question of being an object. He is less interested in anxiety and the other as a moralizing tale on loving well and focuses instead on the threat anxiety poses to our sense of separation, which is integral to a sense of vitality.

Lacan sees in the series of lost objects—breast, feces, phallus, gaze, voice—a point of identification (to be sucked, shat, fucked, exposed, spoken). There is a strange bidirectional movement: we have to allow ourselves to be these things (why not, it's enjoyable), yet we also have to break the absolute identification with the object. To be sucked or fucked is momentary, not absolute. Through a consideration of this detachable, partial object that is enjoyed, the one highlighted by Freud in his theory of sexuality, Lacan locates a classic trope of hysteria.

In one passage, Lacan considers the idea of one's arm, which, if it is a symbol of one's will, could become an object under threat. Someone could seize control of it, like when they call you their right-hand man. Or we could leave it behind on the metro or in our analyst's waiting room, like an ordinary umbrella: "We analysts know what that means.

The experience of the hysteric is significant enough to know that this comparison, which affords a glimpse of the fact that an arm can be forgotten, neither more or less than a mechanical arm, is no forced metaphor" (Lacan 2014, 217). What Lacan means to show is that anxiety, especially castration anxiety, is not only a question of dismemberment and bodily harm. It is also the recognition of the unconscious in all this psychopathology of everyday life, including the cornerstone of loss—the realization that we are not masters of our own bodies.

Lacan concludes that not controlling one's arm could be reassuring because if I don't have it, then no one else does either. It is not a question of absolute control, self-mastery, or being out of control and about to be dismembered—a discourse every analyst will recognize immediately in the oscillation of patients' anxiety. All the platitudes concerning letting go, including those steps involved in giving oneself over to a higher power, file in. These are not wrong. But in their simplicity they miss what is more radical about the unconscious and the sexual relation to the object: the necessity of conversion for the transformation of anxiety.

Anxiety arises in liminal spaces, in the sensation of oneself as a body in relation to something outside, the sense of a foreign edge. Scratch the surface of anxiety, and you will find an agoraphobia that eventually betrays the unconscious as it acts upon the patient. Action, when based in anxiety, is reduced to controlling the appearance of this Otherness, either in oneself or the other person. Here we get a glimpse of why anxiety must be tied to sexuality. Regression for Lacan is regression away from the recognition of separation, calling up earlier phantasmatic modes of enjoyment, provoking the anxiety that wants to grind this sexual unconscious to a halt. For Lacan, the meaning of separation is not "this is my arm and that is yours, my arm does what I want it to" but instead something more like "who knows whose arms any of these are, all the same, I'm doing just fine, it's not going to come off if my attention lapses." Separation happens despite the lack of any firm outlines, not because of them. Separation is not an indulgence in an individual sense of boundaries or achieved autonomy; rather, separation is what it means to have a relationship with one's unconscious.

Lacan pushes this point even further when he states that separation is the lack of any common satisfaction whatsoever. This is made the most apparent by the idea of *coitus interruptus* not as the failure to orgasm but rather as the failure to achieve common satisfaction, which only further marks our separation. In an interrupted enjoyment, the body feels the other's pulling out or pulling away, before any "conclusion" is reached—namely, the sexual nonrelation. What appears in *coitus interruptus* is the embodiment of castration. This is why it is named as *the* source of anxiety by Freud. Lacan concurs with psychoanalysis supposedly at its worst, uniting, in his unique and paradoxical way, the early and late theory of Freud: "Thanks to Freud, we have this cleaving point in our grasp. This in itself is miraculous" (168).

We have the separation between sexual partners and also the separation between the anatomical organ—in this case the penis—and orgasm or ejaculation. One is stripped away as the other emerges, most concretely, in the penis's detumescence.

> I'll simply say that anxiety is promoted by Freud in its quintessential function right where the accompaniment to orgasmic buildup is precisely uncoupled from the engagement of the instrument. The subject may well be reaching ejaculation, but it's an ejaculation on the outside, and anxiety is provoked by the sidelining of the instrument in *jouissance*. Subjectivity is focalized in the falling-away of the phallus.
>
> (168)

This passage is fascinating for the constellation of terms of separation—uncoupled, sidelined, falling away—turning around the "deciduous" (168) character of the object.

Separation is thus not simply about the imaginary violence done to a mother's body, nor the imaginary violence of the child's ejection from it, nor even guilt about sexual enjoyment, but simply a fact of the individual's separateness, which manages to escape our notice, especially when it concerns the phallus. Escapes, that is, except when we are anxious in the face of so much *coitus interruptus*.

Perhaps this helps us understand why anxiety is the only real or true emotion for Lacan; this moment of facing a certain reality, being signaled to it. If one can make it to the other side of anxiety, then the rest of the emotions—always sexual, always labile, like love, hate, disgust, and ignorance—can emerge in this changed economy of desire. *Coitus interruptus* (and the theory of anxiety, then) is no joke. The figure of interruption, like the most powerful day residue found in incomplete acts, sets up the dream and helps us think desire and the body, materiality and language, together.

WHAT THERE IS

Lacan's musings on Freud's theory of *coitus interruptus and separation* also open the door to a nonphallic sexuality and a different configuration of the relationship between anxiety and enjoyment. It is important to note that these intimations around female sexuality are well before the conclusions wrought in the infamous 1972–1973 Seminar XX, concerning *la langue* and surplus *jouissance*. In Lacan's reading of Freud's obsession with *coitus interruptus*, he sees not some silly, overly biological redundancy nor even some misguided sociological commentary but instead this fascinating place where psyche forms in a border space: in between two bodies, in between the somatic and phantasmatic expectations, in between anxiety and conversion, aroused by a sexual relationship that encounters the fall or loss of the object.

Lacan's Seminar X, *Anxiety* (2014), focuses on our relationship to the deciduous object. The emphasis is on the object as objectal, as opposed to any idea of objectivity. The object drags us along, the supposed autonomy of the subject increasingly abolished in this drift. At this edge, we might find a point of equilibrium, inside and outside being established through what Lacan calls a circumcision in the economy of desire, enacted through separation. A separation must take place at the furthest and most foreign edge of ourselves, in contact with what is absolutely Other. He uses the surreal naturalistic fable of a shrimp that needs to imbibe a grain of sand to establish equilibrium.

The shrimp, he says, needs to take this outside inside. But it has to be the right grain of sand—scientists made them swallow all kinds of things that set them off balance, including grains of metal that allowed the scientists to play with these poor little shrimp using magnets. Strange that evolution can make room for something like the shock of birth, not as the separation from the mother's body but as this foreign exterior (oxygen, breath) invading us from the outside. Separation, then, is an achievement, even when it is a fact. Separation is always the separation of my body and yours, establishing any sense we might begin to have of an inside and outside. It is up to psychoanalysis, he says, to do an exhaustive study of this frontier.

What is important here is fundamentally counterintuitive, even counter to the sense we like to have of what Lacan is on about. In this tale of anxiety, there is very little about the metaphoric nature of the subject, nor even the subject of desire. Instead, what we find is the syncope of the subject in an anxiety that finally pulls them to the edge of themselves. There is no constitution of desire without this anxiety and without the work of traversing anxiety. Women, Lacan claims, are much better at bearing this movement through anxiety. Men—especially when it comes to detumescence and castration anxiety—are in much worse shape.

Freud marveled at how well a woman can live with frigidity or sexual failure, whereas for men, impotence often destroys them. Lacan seems to concur with Freud's conclusion that men are more prone to neurasthenia, which often leads to more hysterical women. These hysterical women—whose anxiety folds easily into desire—should, according to Lacan, make better analysts. They have within their grasp the importance of the desire of the analyst for conducting an analysis, including being able to navigate the waters of countertransference and resisting the anxiety of patients, which can ensnare you.

Taking up the question of the end of analysis as a confrontation with castration, Lacan says that if one looks at the question of anxiety we might understand how analysis ends up "in this dead end whereby the negative that stamps the physiological function of copulation in the human being finds itself promoted to the level of the subject in the form of an irreducible lack" (176). The confrontation with the bedrock refusal of castration is the key to ending analysis, whose end, then, is like the end of sex, the end of tumescence—and who would want that?

Is this negative stamp of the physiological function of copulation really what surges up at the end of analysis? Is this what Freud was after in naming *coitus interruptus* the source of anxiety? Is Lacan as ridiculous as Freud in these speculations?

Lacan's conclusions follow Freud: "no desire can be fulfilled without castration. To the extent that *jouissance* is involved, that is that she has my Being in her sights, woman can only reach it by castrating me" (180–81). He continues, mimicking Freud's despair by imputing it to his listeners: "May this not lead the male portion of my audience into any resignation with regard to the ever-palpable effects of this basic truth in what is called, using a classificatory term, conjugal life" (181). The effects on marriage are palpable for both sexes. However, Lacan carries on, for the women, how can we not see that when it comes to castration anxiety they are lacking nothing—she is already castrated, so to speak—and it's the other who has to bear its effects, which she would like very much because it would return her desire to her? "The fact is that on this point she has nothing wanting" because she wants everything from the position that she holds (181). In wanting this penis, perhaps, he muses, what she wants is for the other to be able to tolerate the castration implied in having a sexual relationship, so that, for once, her desire can meet with another desire. This is Lacan's affirmative reading of female desire.

What the woman is, Lacan says, is more real and more true. None of this ultimately resolves the question of her desire nor the question of her anxiety—she has trouble with it in her own right—but in the end, Lacan is at pains to say she is not lacking even if she is wanting, and this margin gives room to her desire in a fascinating way, in not having to bear the organ and the gap between it as instrument, deciduous object, and *jouissance*. Lacan can place her differently in relation not only to what she is but all that is.

So much so, that the fact of wanting does not unravel her because taking an interest in the object entails far fewer, as he puts it, complications for her. The object does not need to fill a lack in her; the object is additive, a surplus, like the grain of sand to the shrimp. Lacan insists that there is something truly original here. In saying it, he feels this is the only way to unravel something about the nature of penis envy that has haunted psychoanalysis as a deadlock since Freud wrote "Analysis Terminable and Interminable" (1937).

To elucidate this, Lacan goes on to provide a fascinating case, one of the few of his own that he spoke of in any detail. He begins, "One day a woman tells me that her husband, whose insistences are, if I may, part and parcel of the foundation of the marriage, leaves her alone a little too long for her not to notice. . . . This is when she comes out with a sentence. . . . She exposes herself as follows—*small matter whether he desires me, provided he doesn't desire others*" (187–88). Lacan says that he won't say that this is commonplace—something about a woman's jealousy or possessiveness or whatever—but that we can only really understand it from the constellation of what follows, especially as regards the statement as a message from within the transference.

The withdrawal of the husband's insistences, an attention that sustains her, including a complaint regarding his clumsiness, opens up a field of desire. Lacan says she suddenly begins to speak with a peculiar precision about her state, one that shows that tumescence isn't simply the privilege of the man:

> This woman, whose sexuality is quite normal, bears witness to what occurs for her if, when she is driving, for example, an alert flashes up for a moving entity that makes her say to herself something along the lines of *God, a car!* Well, inexplicably, she notices the existence of a vaginal swelling. This is what strikes her that day and she notes that, during some periods, the phenomenon will occur when just any old object comes into her visual field, to all appearances utterly foreign to anything of a sexual nature.
>
> (188)

This woman's desirous gaze is returned to her through the withdrawal of her husband's. Any old object can become the trigger for an experience of *jouissance* that arises like a flash, a signal, as the other face of anxiety. The state, she goes on to say, stops of its own accord—it has a rhythm all its own; it begins and ends by surprise, a kind of bodily symphony in relation to the world.

This is the limit of the analogy with the man, for her tumescence does not follow the same path from tumescence to detumescence. Rather, it transfers onto a whole field of objects and then stops as abruptly as it started. It is a tolerable cutoff point, or a cut that is tolerated, in particular because she can bring these observations back to Lacan in her analysis. This leads the patient to speak to the peculiarities of the nature of their analytic relationship:

> Each of her initiatives are dedicated to me, her analyst. *I can't say devoted*, she adds, *that would mean it was done with a certain aim, but no, any old object forces me to evoke you as a witness, not even to have your approval of what I see, no, simply your gaze, and in saying that, I'm going slightly too far, let's say that this gaze helps me to make each thing assume meaning.*
>
> (188)

What we see is that this object that enters into her sight and evokes a feeling of vaginal excitement is linked in some way to the function of the gaze in the transference, which renders, as witness, what she sees as meaningful. This is not the demanding clumsy gaze of her husband nor even her desirous looking (especially looking for Lacan's approval) but something about the analyst as witness, the one who can be evoked as watching this emergence of desire in a field that surrounds her. This object can be any old thing, but in this there is a pivot between assumed meaning (or the object as desired by the other for its place or meaning in relation to *her* desire—what Lacan would call a bad caricature of psychoanalysis) and *jouissance*. This is the circuit that the other is used to support. All of this is prefaced by a separation, a fact—her husband's leaving her alone a little too long—which sets off the session and this series of confessions.

Lacan carries on with his description of the session. She has an association to Steve Passeur's play *Je vivrai un grand amour*, which leads her to speak about falling in love with her husband and then about her first love. She says about this first love that she enveloped herself in a series of lies, like a cocoon, in order to be exactly what she wanted to be in his eyes. This gesture is not exactly one done for his gaze but rather to support her own in relation to a first love. She ties this moment to the transference to Lacan, showing the difference between this first love and what is now happening:

> What I strive to be here with you is quite the opposite. I strive always to be truthful with you. I'm not writing a novel with you. I write it when I'm not with you. She comes back to the threading, still stitch by stitch, of this dedicating of each gesture, which is not necessarily a gesture supposed to please me, nor one that would necessarily be in conformity with my thinking. You can't say she was forcing her talent [for lying].
> (188–89)

She does not make herself into what he wants to see but what she wants to see about herself, this act dedicated to Lacan.

With that, she comes back to what she does with Lacan, which, he notes, is very different from this configuration of first love: "After all, what she wanted was not so much for me to look at her as for my gaze to replace hers. *I appeal to the assistance of your person. The gaze, my gaze, is insufficient when it comes to capturing everything that stands to be absorbed from the outside. It's not about watching me do something, it's about doing it for me*" (189). I find this moment absolutely beautiful, this idea of an appeal for assistance in order to capture the everything that can be taken in from the outside. The insufficiency of one when it comes to the desire for this absorption.

It is not the strategy of first love, where the other, this fiction, props her up and allows her to exist, but something else more desirous. The relationship with Lacan is another iteration of the question of the gaze,[4] but this time she finds in her transference a support that allows her to see the everything that is there for the taking. She is not taking the other in, duping them, nor is she taken in by her own ideal; rather, she allows her gaze to drop by replacing it with her analyst's eyes, and it is through this falling away that the world flares up—God, a car!

There is a funny question of *who goes too far* that circulates between Lacan and this patient in the attempt to characterize their relationship;

both seem to return the question to the other again and again, trying to find the right angle. Lacan characterizes her desire by saying that it's not about his looking at her—certainly it isn't—but rather that it's a matter of his gaze replacing hers. But replacement is his word, and she corrects him. It is more about assistance, dedication, assumption, witnessing—calling upon this other set of eyes in order to allow or frame this space where any object can be a source of desire, a great love to live, a literal swelling in her surroundings.

Her eyes are returned to her at the moment where the object appears in its intensity as a source of excitement, differentiated from an indifferent surround. This witnessing provides a possible assumption of meaning through the other, but this meaning is just meaningfulness in and of itself, meaning that it is not and never will be, a meaning specifically addressed to the other's gaze or what this gaze is imputed to want.

Not approval, as she says, but simply an indication of herself as wanting in this sheer metonymy of objects. It causes these objects to flash up simultaneously with some movement in her own body. This wanting seems to need, at bottom, the encounter with another that can want in kind, that can hold this place—without either attaching themselves to anything in particular. Is this not the very essence of transference love? Especially an idea of transference love as work? And is this not what it means to encounter another who is without anxiety, especially castration anxiety? Lacan does not say it, but I think the implication is there.

Any "common satisfaction" is dependent upon some realized separation, which raises the question of what is common. What we see in the case is that by dispensing with her gaze or letting it fall, she calls on the analyst (as a support, as a supplement) in order to make the object of her enjoyment appear. Is this the same deciduous object that is embodied negatively in the anxiety of *coitus interruptus*? Or is the object transformed when it is not the anxious signal of separation but the voluptuous consequence of it? Lacan ends this clinical vignette contesting her use of the term "remote controlled," which he says is in poor taste:

> *I am*, she says, *remote controlled*. This does not express any metaphor and there is no *sentiment d'influence*, believe me, no feeling of being

influenced. I'm only isolating this formula because you may have read it in the papers in connection with that left-wing politician who, after getting embroiled in a staged shooting, thought he ought to give us the immortal example of how, in politics, the left is always effectively remote-controlled by the right. Moreover, that's precisely how a tight relation of equal representation can be set up between the two sides.

(189)

I'm not entirely convinced that she exercises such poor taste in her choice of words—after all, the distance between the screen and the remote feels right, or the remote as double to a function already contained in the device it controls, to say nothing of the additive object that this remote is in itself.

Nevertheless, what Lacan is at pains to argue on behalf of his patient is that what she is speaking about isn't about any reciprocity or reciprocal relationship, like the symbiotic nature of a two-party political system. It is something else. The transference is not the establishment of reciprocity but the possibility that arises from the achievement of separation. The relationship establishes an asymmetry that lends itself to the support the patient can find through the analyst. This allows the object to act as a supplement and not as a negative, anxiety-inducing cipher.

"So, where is all this leading us? To the vessel. Is the female vessel empty or full? It matters not because it is sufficient unto itself, even if it is to be *consummated stupidly*, as my patient puts it" (189). Lacan returns to the idea that for the female nothing is lacking, nothing is wanting. What this means is that the object is not called on to fill in for a lack, nor is it desired on the basis of some lack—the supposed penis envy—but rather that it is a surplus: "the presence of the object is an extra" (189). Why? Lacan says, it is not bound to the "lack of the object cause of desire, to the $(-\varphi)$ to which it is bound in men" (189). Men have anxiety, he says, about not being able, and women are something that fills in for what is missing—hence the woman as phallus for the man. What matters to us here is "to grasp the woman's bond to the infinite possibilities or rather indeterminate possibilities of desire in the field that stretches out around her," namely, this everything that stands to be absorbed from the outside (189). Infinite and indeterminate—this is a truth about the object as sexual for Freud, something that Lacan here links to female sexuality in particular.

Her anxiety, Lacan says, is only the anxiety faced with the desire of the Other, and at the end of the day, who knows what this Other covers over—Lacan will not engage in a quest for origins. In any case, this matters little if the analysis comes to the point where she can awaken this object through the Other for her pleasure. "She tempts herself by tempting the Other," and, as the famous story goes, she can tempt with just about anything: "It so happens that this apple was already good enough, little fish that it was, to hook the angler. The desire of the Other is what interests her" insofar as it can come to support any old thing, any little fish or apple of her choosing (190).

For the man, on the other hand, things are the other way around; desire is a cover for anxiety, and *jouissance* is sustained in a close relation to anxiety—something that leads to all kinds of complications, from idealization and debasement in the sphere of love to the half-pleasures of interruption, spoiling, and feeling forced. Desire and *jouissance* pull against each other at this hinge of anxiety, with little room for transformation. Here, Lacan says, "you can see the margin he still has to cover to be in range of *jouissance*"—as if he can barely find this edge or evoke this object through the Other to make of it something at a distance from himself (190). The woman is often soldered to him, like Lacan's patient's pestering husband. And there is always an imposture in the realm of male desire, meaning that he is posing, wrapping himself in a cocoon, a fictional envelope—like our patient with her first love—here, made from the fibers of the woman whom he claims as part of himself.

Letting desire be seen from within these wrappings is often a source of massive anxiety, a moment of unveiling. For Lacan's patient, the question of letting it be seen is precisely what is played with. In fact, this is where she finds her greatest pleasure:

> There isn't only showing and seeing, there is also *letting something be seen*. For women, whose danger at the very most comes from the masquerade, the something that is there to be let seen is what there is. Of

course, if there's not much, it's anxiety provoking, but it's still what there is, whereas for men, letting their desire be seen essentially amounts to letting what there is not, be seen.

(191)

I find this moment in the seminar fascinating. Not only is desire a question of any object whatsoever—this infinite surplus relationship to the object world—but it also hinges on a relationship of what there is, not what there is not.

This "what there is" is intransitive in relation to the Other—making oneself seen, heard, sucked, and so on through temptation—using them to extract these precious nothings, these objects that open one's access to an infinite field of pleasure, if not love. It merely means having to let what is there reveal itself, to know the worth of crossing the threshold of anxiety—something indispensable for psychoanalysis. It is not a question of the object as what is lacking or lost but simply of revealing what is there and allowing the object to become this additive enjoyment, this surplus pleasure.

If psychoanalysis has tended to emphasize the internal world, subjectivity, and lack or loss, here Lacan reverses this almost entirely. He concludes this section addressing the men: "so, you see, don't believe that this situation, whose demonstration might strike you as fairly complex, is for all that to be taken as something especially desperate. Though it most certainly doesn't represent it as something easy, can you fail to spot the access to *jouissance* that it opens for the man?" (191). Lacan is suddenly less pessimistic than Freud, even less pessimistic than the recurring characterization of Lacan's announcement of the absence of the sexual relationship.

Here, Lacan shows that somewhere, namely, on the side of the object, we can see the point of access. Lacan will go on to call on psychoanalysts for an exhaustive catalogue of the frontier where anxiety meets with the possible appearance of the object—what he calls the cutoff point where the deciduous nature of the object reveals itself. Crossing this threshold means being able to reconfigure anxiety and enjoyment in new, surprising ways, something Lacan would go on to elaborate much later with his notion of the "sinthome" (2017).

Being able to write or rewrite something fundamental in our relationship to the body is certainly something that we can see in the language of the circumcision of the heart in Christian theology, linking religious and psychoanalytic conversion:

> Admittedly people say—*I want your heart and nothing more.* By that, they mean to designate goodness knows what spiritual something or other, the essence of your Being, or even your love. But, here as always, language betrays the truth. . . . In the formula, I want your heart . . . as in any metaphor of an organ, the heart is to be taken to the letter. It functions as a part of the body, as, if I may say, part of the innards.
>
> (2014, 216)

The anxiety of being the object of desire must be seen as literal, read to the letter—*I want your heart.* I want your organ. I want to be the organ of your enjoyment. Desire, Lacan reminds us, is always the desire for a body. The problem, of course, is that these bodies or organs will always remain utterly separate—a desiring machine without a subject, a surplus of indeterminate objects outside of any narrative. "If what is most me lies on the outside, not because I projected it there but because it was cut off from me," he writes, "the paths I shall take to retrieve it afford an altogether different variety" (223).

The conversion of anxiety is critical. Not only is it the transformation of the superegoic gaze, but it is also the opening up of a different kind of object relationship altogether, to say nothing of the transformation in the relationship to pleasure and sexuality. The consequences for psychoanalysis seem vast, seem to compose an altogether different system and map than what typically transpires as its most basic coordinates. Is it a question of psychoanalysis as a passage to the outside, an object-oriented psychoanalysis that jettisons any idea of "interior" life and even the coordinates of subjectivity, especially insofar as they rely on this inwardness?

In the case of Lacan's patient in particular, we see a strange functionality arising between them, like two bodies humming, a woman without eyes, an analyst without a body, and an object given all the life there is to give between the two so that something can flash up before her eyes, from him to her and back again. The world is suddenly an infinite meaningful field without, for all that, taking on any particular narrative. That was the problem with first love, with the coordinates of the gaze, with the fiction that she wrapped herself in. This gaze dropped, in handing herself over to her indeterminate analyst's eyes, she finds this infinite possibility in the world around her. And is this not what Lacan feels a woman has always wanted—the whole world and nothing more?

VIII

THREE VISIONS OF PSYCHOANALYSIS

The body is the unconscious: seeds of ancestors sequenced in its cells, and mineral salts consumed, and mollusks caressed, broken bits of wood, and worms feasting on its cadaver underground, or else the flame that incinerates it and the ash it yields, epitomizing it in impalpable powder, and the people, plants, and animals whose paths it crosses and with whom it rubs shoulders, and the tales from long-gone nurses, and monuments in ruins covered with lichens, and enormous turbines in factories fabricating extraordinary alloys from which its prosthetic devices will be made, and rough or lisping phonemes, with which its tongue makes spoken noises, and laws engraved on steles, and a secret desire for murder or immortality. The body touches on everything with the secret tip of its bony fingers. And everything ends up making a body, down to the very corpus *of dust assembling and dancing a vibrant dance in the thin streak of light where the last day of the world draws to a close.*

—JEAN-LUC NANCY, *CORPUS*

THREE VISIONS OF PSYCHOANALYSIS

Psychoanalysis has increasingly traded on the figures of identity and interior depth—its task reduced to the epithet "know thyself." The analyst, like Virgil, escorts the patient down through the layers of hell so that he or she can emerge changed. How can one be at odds with such classical images?

I am more and more weary of these figures, these tired clichés, the tasks as they have been handed down to me. There has to be another way of thinking about the subject—to think about the psyche while refusing to re-evoke, yet again, the trope of what is "on the inside." Identity and interiority feel like versions of mastery deployed by those who would like to still their bodies, to form a flat surface. I have a desperate feeling that these concepts have led psychoanalysis seriously astray.

Lacan, of course, in his very particular reading of Freud, tries to do away with them or, at the very least, to make them the outposts of fantasy. We run, he says, headfirst into the wall of epistemological queries concerning what can be known not simply about identity or the mind but also about how we conceive of knowledge or knowing in relation to them. It is not simply a question of how we know what we know about the mind, the body, and the self but how we envision what we think they know or are supposed to know and how. This leads Lacan further and further away from knowledge, sense, and meaning—uprooting any primacy of place it might hold in psychoanalysis (Fink 2013). In any case, the misrecognition runs deep. Deeper than you think.

Present-day psychology—neuroscience, the empire of therapies—trades on different visions of the relationship between knowledge and a body, not only establishing a certain kind of doctor—so regal, so well informed, so clean—but also his object, which is often an identity to be consolidated, a depth to be plumbed and exposed, or a body that should be rendered seamless or declared out of order. I would like to find a different vision of psychoanalysis, or a different vision in psychoanalysis itself, one that finds a way to stop this machine and open into another territory—a territory that speaks the body more than speaks about it, a territory where the outside, or the external, isn't a derogatory term implying some Valhalla has been achieved through the twenty-first-century psychological subject—certainly it hasn't. I would like to find a vision of psychoanalysis that gives room to this body without lapsing into banalities. This is, of course, the territory that this book is trying to map with the term "conversion." Through the strange mediums of fire, touch, and madness—a meditation on three thinkers, like three cases, Bachelard, Nancy, Foucault—I will begin to define the terrain of psychoanalysis differently.

Each, in his own way, points to an exteriority that is both a sexual form and an object, changing the place or means of meeting the psychoanalyst. Each evokes the object of psychoanalysis and highlights different aspects of conversion, from the antimetaphoric question of substance in Bachelard, whose love for fire as the first object brings to the surface the question of chemical combustion and conversion; to Nancy, who evokes the body neither as spiritual nor imaginary but as something that blocks sense and brings separation to bear; and, finally, to Foucault, who makes conversion a question of the outside of language by imagining a future where discourse ceases to be mad and so will fail to convert anything, forcing us to place our bets on mad language over rationality. These three meditations will be quick. Hold on to your hats.

THE PSYCHOANALYSIS OF FIRE

The philosopher Bachelard, writing in the 1930s and 1940s, declares that he wants to deobjectify the body, to remove from the body all objects, in order "to free it from the narcissism caused by the first contact with the object" (Bachelard 1964, 4). This first object is in fact an antiobject—pure surplus, movement, excess, and therefore not static nor sedimented into an image. It precedes narcissism and potentially undoes it.[1] It is, he says, best embodied by fire, always already stolen and coveted, fire whose interior we cannot examine with a body, whose interior is never given. To get closer to this primal object, we must give body to fire or flames—give the substance of flames to thought—not the reverse, since conceptualizing fire would be to render it, once again, static. Conceptualizing fire is to form it into the image we would like to have of ourselves. The work of fire, he claims, would cure the mind of its happy illusions—cure the thirst for the knowledge of fire, for insight into combustible bodies, for the endless quest for an image. One can read in Bachelard the attempt to construct the coordinates of a self-conversion. Contra any epistemological quest, we need, says Bachelard, a psychoanalysis of fire.

His book begins with a warning: this work will in no way have increased your knowledge. "Turning inwards upon ourselves we turn aside from truth. When we carry out inner experiments, we inevitably contradict objective experiment" (5). This psychoanalysis of substances, fire, no less than blood, water, earth, or air, "could demonstrate human error, the clear demonstration of how the fascination exerted by the object *distorts induction*" (5). Bachelard, who was a scientist first, has very little faith in turning inward, yet he acknowledges how difficult it is to view the world, how distorted it is by human fantasy and fascination. The question of substance, the most basic substances in the world around us, and the almost deconstructive work of psychoanalysis together might reveal some piece of the universe. He says this as if this has always been the task of scientists—to psychoanalyze themselves first, then theorize second.

To the Oedipal complex—the myth of civilization par excellence in the cooling form of family and territoriality—Bachelard says we must add the Novalis complex, the fire-world of unfallen life, the fires of pre-creation, as well as the Empedocles complex, the destruction of the world by fire, the self-consuming flames of the Last Judgment. Fire demands respect, a respect for life and respect for the end of life. This lesson is communicated to children through fire, what he calls social interdiction as our first general knowledge of fire—don't touch it, it's hot!—making the prohibition on touching fire the first moment of splitting between the intellectual and the physical: "fire, then, can strike without having to burn . . . the blow of the ruler is replaced by the angry voice; the angry voice by the recital of the dangers of fire, by the legends concerning fire from heaven" (11). When the natural, meaning the substances, are mixed with the social, we have the beginning of prejudiced knowledge. Why? Because the knowledge of fire is transformed into the arduous desire for knowledge drawn into a Promethean will to catch up with the knowledge of fathers and overturn their interdictions by disobedience or acquisition. The life of the intellect will have no other substratum than this distorted rivalry.

For Freud, fire was invented not in order to forge iron, cook, or keep warm but rather in order to urinate on it—an alarming conclusion that lays bare the strangeness of psychoanalytic deduction. What the psychoanalysis of fire demonstrates is not simply the sexualization of fire, nor even mere burning ambition and its inhibition, but how the conquest of what is superfluous in a familial war holds greater power than anything seemingly necessary. The object as surplus and excess is more important than the object as a product, especially as an object of knowledge. We should return to fire for fire's sake, return fire to fire—this is why the final flames of destruction, the last judgment, promise renewal more than progressive change or the development of any object for utility.

Empedoclean reveries of fire, like the dream of a burning child, make the ever-present call for a final sacrifice heard—envelop me, let me meet my destiny and leave without a trace. "If fire, which, after all, is quite an exceptional and rare phenomenon, was taken to be a constituent element of the Universe, is it not because it is an element of human thought, the prime element of reverie?" (18). Fire is the beginning and end of all reverie. None of these musings, Bachelard points out again, has any basis in objective reality through some means of observation. We cannot see this work of fire in human psychology or civilization. Yet does it not remain profoundly real? More real than supposed reality? Has it not always been the most active element? This is why it is given such a prime place in reverie or is seen as reverie itself, this original burning. It is a dream of substance, or, even better, it is the substance of dream. Fire always returns us to fire. Because of this, "the dream," Bachelard concludes, "is stronger than experience" (20).

In these reflections on fire it is important to grasp that Bachelard does not see this as a means of moving from reality to metaphor. He is no Jungian. In fact, his claim is that we are increasingly moving in the reverse direction, from metaphor to reality—"it is this absurdity which explains the discovery of fire" (37). Myths of fire move from subjective origins toward reality: the fire hidden within the human body is the origin of real fire; fire explains the colors of birds or earth. Not vice versa. Fire creates material experiences, hypnotic details of substance, emerging from somatic and affective life, away from knowledge and codified language. Fire resists sight and touch, and in the intuition of inner heat, the dream of going into an interior without interior is born. We move to the center of an image in order to return the image to substance, searching for an authenticity the image bartered away. For Bachelard, fire drains all sentimental or realist pathos from understanding, crashing through the traps of narcissism and the hubris of knowledge.

Nothing could be more sexual than this work of fire, or, rather, this is the substance of sexuality. Yet Bachelard suddenly concludes that this sexualized fire cannot be equated with a sexual relationship, neither with procreation (seed and spark) nor with any reduction of the problem to a stupid tautology: fire is life and life is fire. The naïve lover's dream, the romantic soldering of sex and procreation, or sex and life, needs to return to the psychoanalysis of fire to challenge itself—not only its idealism but its materialism as well. Thinking for Bachelard cannot reside in any naturalism or biologism that wants to do away with the subjective in the name of an easy objectivity—for nothing is more infused with fantasy than science for Bachelard, who deconstructs its many iterations to show them as nothing more than a sexual reverie. On the other hand, Bachelard is neither a romantic nor an idealist, which always runs into both the wall of material reality and the human proclivity to wish and dream in a way that pronounces upon the world: "'I am manipulating,' says the alchemist. 'No, you are dreaming.' 'I am dreaming,' says Novalis. 'No, you are manipulating'" (55). Psychoanalysis, for Bachelard, is poised to take on this problem.

The psychoanalysis of fire wants to reach back behind the desire for knowledge and the desire for love that is behind it. The changes wrought by fire cannot be simply material or ideal; they are changes in substance, pure movement, the play of forces. "Through fire everything changes.

And when we want everything to change we call on fire" (57). The dream of love is soldered to the value of creation; fire is set against this, moving in the direction of destruction, even if it is renewal. Both death and resurrection, for Bachelard, must be without any particular value—not even the transvaluation of value.

It is simply the value of transformation—or perhaps better, the value of substance—that the psychoanalysis of fire values as the only proof of existence and its continuation: endless conversion and combustion, infinite fire. By turning away from the idealization of fire—against fire metaphorically used to think of love or birth or even death—toward fire for fire's sake, Bachelard feels he has worn out the patience of his reader. He adds to his work a second warning and a surprising address to his audience regarding his own writing. He states toward the end of this strange book: "this impatience in itself is a sign; we would like the realm of values to be a closed realm. We would like to judge values without bothering about the primary empirical meanings" (106). The in-mixing of fact and value will be left behind in flames or force alone.

PSYCHOANALYSIS OF TOUCH

To the sign of "this impatience" by Bachelard we will add Jean-Luc Nancy's "this is my body." For Nancy, the obsession with showing a "this" in "this is my body" lends itself as much to a few jokes as does fire, since the desired "this"—this substance, this body—can never show itself with any certainty, while it is nevertheless certainly there. Saying so—this is my body—is some strange additive. Trying to hold the thing forth is at best an awkward redundancy. The assertion "this!" is purely comical. "Sensory certitude, as soon as it is touched, turns into chaos, a storm where all sense runs wild. Body is certitude shattered and blown to bits" (Nancy 2008, 5). What can "this" be?

Nancy calls the familiar strangeness of "this" in "this is my body" the nonmelancholic agony of nakedness, of being laid open and touched. If we are going to write about the body, it cannot be a discourse on appearance or spectacle, on the imaginary body or body as phantasm, nor can it be a hymn to immediacy or some uninterrupted real to be unveiled, as if the *this* was simply possible, even in a reachable beyond. Nancy states in no uncertain terms that these are religious iterations of incarnation in the model of the image—always empty or full, spiritual or disembodied. We should be wary of metaphorizing what is essentially concrete.

No access is granted to the body; still, the body is open. What never asks to be deciphered is what defines opening as space, spatial. Neither full nor empty but this, there: "it is a skin, variously folded, refolded, unfolded, multiplied, invaginated, exogastrulated, orificed, evasive, invaded, stretched, relaxed, excited, distressed, tied, untied. In these and a thousand other ways, the body makes room for existence" (15). With Nancy, "this" body will not lead to a discourse on the ineffable, on the silent mysteries linking the body again with the spiritual. There is no "sense" when it comes to bodies. Yet the non-sense of the sensory is neither the estimation of the sublime, nor the negative coloring of absurdity, nor the contortions of knowledge. The non-sense of the body is a place of clarity in the sense of something shining and distinct rather than lucid—a brilliance of difference.

The body, Nancy says, demands other categories of force and thought, ones that manage to touch at the limit the "this" of some singular body— "touching the body with the incorporeality of 'sense'" (11). How could this touching of the body with incorporeal sense even be possible? Bodies, he tells us, are addressed to one another: they are "existence addressed to an outside," like lovers (11). In the thought of bodies is the purest of separations, namely, the separation or cut between bodies that gives form to love as address, touch—"it's the separation of substances which alone allows them their singular chance" (19). Touch, here, is the overriding concern because it is about difference, touching difference, the attempt to cross a chasm, to affirm and overcome separation at once.

The exscription of bodies is evoked for Nancy by Freud in what he calls his "most fascinating and perhaps (I say this without exaggerating) most decisive statement," which appears in a posthumous note: "*Psyche ist ausgedehnt: weiss nichts davon.*" "The psyche's extended: knows nothing about it" (21). Nancy explains this: "The 'psyche,' in other words, is body, and this is precisely what escapes it, and its escape (we may suppose), or its process of escape, constitutes it as 'psyche,' in a dimension of not (being able/wanting)-to-know-itself" (21). This exteriorization maps a terrain beyond sense—a territoriality or *topos* of tensions—where a psychoanalysis of touch might take shape because of this psyche that cannot know itself for what it is. So it must touch itself there.

Nancy points to a crucial part of Freud's vision of the body in *Three Essays on the Theory of Sexuality* ([1905c] 1995), where the question of the unconscious is much closer to a sexual terrain that could be described ruthlessly in bodily terms—zonal tensions, pain-pleasure, stimulation, substitutes—while the ego remains merely the projection of this body's surface extended, exteriorized, and having to know nothing about it. How, then, did the unconscious come to be thought in terms of interior, depth, inside, and even eventually in terms of sense or signification?

> It's even more surprising then, that a certain psychoanalytic discourse would seem to insist, while denying its object, on making the body "signify," rather than flushing out signification as something that always screens off the spacing of bodies. This kind of analysis "ectopizes" (or "utopizes") the body beyond-place: it volatilizes it, indexing it to the incorporeality of sense.
>
> (23)

The body is indexed but screened off. Nancy is not saying that the body is without sense—that would be oxymoronic—but that the sense of the body is something other than sense as signification.

We need the body of sense, the touching of body and sense; this can only take place at the limit, which is the meaning of extension, of a not-being-able to know itself there where it encounters something beyond itself. Sense as feeling, against sense as meaning, happens at the place where we make contact with the other. Everything else, Nancy says, volatilizes—making neurosis an effect of disaffected utopias, the language of the untouched, the movement of the unmoved, and the problem of an incorporeal dream. Conversion is perhaps best thought of here as the move from an incorporeal dream to a *corpus*, a body of work and the body as work.

Once Nancy turns to Freud, he is quick to evoke the hysteric as exemplary of this structure. He contests seeing her as a signifying or speaking body, as many would have it, since that would mean no longer being a body. Instead, he wants to see hysteria (and here he moves from the individual to the pathology) as this bodily nonknowledge:

> The body's becoming totally parasitical upon the incorporeality of sense, to the point that it silences incorporeality, thereby showing, in its stead, a piece, a zone, of a-significance. (Because ultimately we would have to know whether the hysteric is engaging mainly in translation and interpretation or in something contrary and much deeper, namely, a resolute blockage of the transmission of sense. Discourse incarnate, or a blocking body: who doesn't see that there is no hysteria without a blocking body?)
>
> (23)

For Nancy, the symptom is deployed in hysteria not in order to convey sense or meaning—to return finally to ideation, understanding taking the place of the once convulsive body—but rather to block sense, to put her body between herself and the other and render sense foreign.

The hysteric shows sense as foreign to this body, hers, with a question about what might be made between them, since bodies—mine and yours—will always retain this distance, this strangeness, this separation, and this antagonism to meaning. The hysteric places her body in relation to the other at the place that blocks the transmission of sense. She finds this point, almost, as it were, unconsciously, knowing nothing about it. And even if nothing gets through—bodies will always remain in their separate places—things do touch. The body touches the other at the place where sense is silenced and perhaps even dismantled. Touching, when this body of sense finally makes itself felt through another. This is what all lover's language concerning the heart—yes, clichéd and rather poor—is meant to convey literally, not metaphorically, being touched or having been.

Nancy's vision of hysteria exalts hysteria and quiets it, giving it an aura of calm. He protects the hysteric, touches her, affirms the limit that her body wants to find in order to be simply what it is:

> The hysterical body is exemplary in its affirmation—at an unattainable limit—of a pure concentration in itself, the pure being-in-itself of its extension, which in turn denies and renders catatonic its extendedness and its spacing . . . this limit manifests the truth of the body, in the form of its implosion. (But perhaps something that opens up in pain or pleasure, and does not withdraw, something that makes room for a passage through the limit, rather than hardening it—is this not, perhaps, a kind of *joyful hysteria*, and the very body of sense?)
>
> (23)

Always the most important thoughts for Nancy are in parentheses at the end of a paragraph, like two distinct halves of a thought touching. Who doesn't see? The psychoanalysts, he seems to be saying. For even if she blocks, implodes, convulses, and resists unfolding or opening in a hardening of her body, like in paralysis, room is nonetheless being given. This is how he reads the hysteric's movements, and from this he states that there is the possibility here of a joyful hysteria. Nancy finds that if you unfold the joy folded in neurotic misery, you will witness the pleasure in pure concentration, density, nerve, as a fidelity to the touch and difference of bodies.

So even if the hysteric puts her body under the sign of withdrawal, she does so as body, not as it is for others as a consequence of ideation. Perhaps she withdraws in order to tease the other, cajole them from their slumber of sense. Finally, Nancy states, "this alone," meaning this hysterical body, "can close or release a space for 'interpretations'" (23). What interpretation? What can be said after this silencing of sense? Nancy is quiet here, leaving us with the thought of the breakthrough of her body and the attempt to say something there and only there. He sees here the figure of writing—etching, more than speaking, the body as opening, exposing, and spacing rather than any stampede or chaos of signification. Whatever happens, it must be the birthing and sharing of bodies, not the incarnation inflating the spiritual life of the sign.

Of course, for Freud, the symptom was the parasitical element of hysteria; the symptom acts like a foreign body, a body implanted within the body, which agitates psyche. Psychoanalysis converts the symptom into the space of analysis—the symptom extending itself ever outward, transforming into the order of the day, the rhythm of analysis. It is here that analyst and patient touch each other. Perhaps we should read this in line with Nancy through the question of bodily extension, this exscription of body as the psychoanalysis of touch. With the psychoanalysis of touch, this act of rhythmic spacing, we have the figures of edge, burn, pain, anguish, and joy instead of meaning and sense. None of this should be aligned with any hysterical *mysterium* or melancholic incorporation but rather be thought about simply as a fact about bodies. The pathos of this kind of signification is precisely what is absent at the limit of the body. It is what is blocked in this joyful and hysterical consenting to the body.

It must be said that this consenting to something that you can never gain access to, never get the sense of, is a kind of madness constituting the double bind of being able neither to speak about it nor keep silent. This anguished joy, says Nancy, is an ordinary madness:

> The madness of the body isn't a crisis, and isn't morbid. It's just this endlessly untied and distended place-taking, tending toward itself. The body's madness is this offering of place . . . there's no crisis, no contortion, no foam, any more than there's room for you and me in the same place at the same time. No secret of the body to be communicated to us, no secret body to be revealed to us.
>
> (59)

This is why he sees this as the draining of neurotic pathos or narcissistic hubris. Instead, the hysteric shows us what it means to keep pressing this body to its outermost edge, to press the body up against speech.

This offering, this injunction—body, madness, press—is all the more urgent when we reflect on the current predicament of bodies in the world, a whole world of bodies, almost eight billion, dense, visible. The body is always already there, hiding in plain sight. How does one even begin to speak about this everywhere excess of body? At one time, it was through the language of sin and the concurrent language of purification. Now, the body, he says, has been saved before it has even arrived—saved for health, for modern medicine and technology, for sport and for pleasure, which only exacerbates the disaster, since this is the pure signification of body, forcing the body to withdraw ever inward, falling into itself, touching nobody.

This divested body mirrors the strange accumulation of body that is ever more disembodied: the singular body becoming anybody in crowds, armies, mass graves and mass murders; the transport of refugees, like so many bodies, across the globe; the billions of images of bodies, ever more indistinct, anonymous, yet there, building up, a surplus of overflowing bodies. This is to say nothing of the accumulation of pornographic displays of bodies, anatomized as zones, parts—which, for Nancy, hides the sexed body as simply the truth of the body in relation to another body.

The body is close to a subject without an object, which is not a subject in the strong sense, since it is so close to itself as objectal. Nancy describes body as weight, as always in the act of weighing—always in relation to its own gravity. The body is an urgency without knowledge, without judgment or value. The body leaves the question of destiny behind because destiny is where everything is weighed in advance, perhaps in order to escape the conundrums of weight, of having a body. Destiny is a dream of weightlessness—what it would be to be disembodied. In life, the press of the body cannot be shaken off. This is the madness. And it is probably the simple truth of separation, which is finally what it means to be this body in this place and to long for or love another.

In the psychoanalysis of touch, the injunctions, values, and vicissitudes of the superego are drained of all ideation. They are reduced to tension, departure, movement, and the thought of touch. This, Nancy says, is what psyche is present to—nothing more, nothing less—not a body to come nor an essential existence, neither a judgment nor a sense of the day, just this permanent press of the body. "Which is why, in this one note by Freud, all of 'psychoanalysis' really has its true program always yet to come" (97). Here, a strange question emerges concerning the institution and program of psychoanalysis—it seems to dictate a program or knowledge that is always to come, that is always deferred. The body is nothing but a "nonknowlege [that] is not a negative knowledge or the negative of knowledge, it's only an absence of knowledge, an absence of the bond," incorporeal, "called 'knowing'" (97). Psychoanalysis is the experience of losing the incorporeality of knowing.

What psychoanalysis knows is only what it touches in an endless transport from one shore to another, this transference as the swerving and turning of bodies—in other words, conversion. Is this not the experience of conversion in analysis—being shaken outside oneself, *res extensa*? This departure of one body for another is one way to think of the psychoanalysis of touch. "This is the world of world-wide departure: the spacing of *partes extra partes*, with nothing to oversee it or sustain it, no Subject for its destiny, taking place only as a prodigious press of bodies" (41). The departure signals an impatience where the possibility of passage that the body offers or affirms is there but can be blocked by sense or meaning, especially when searching for its own meaning.

Psychoanalysis has always been configured as the meeting of minds, or the meeting of words. With Nancy, perhaps we can think of it as this meeting of bodies, subverting the rule of abstinence or, perhaps better, converting it. To screen out the touching of bodies in the framework of meeting, even if in words, is to betray psychoanalysis—the one hope we have for joy.

THE PSYCHOANALYSIS OF MADNESS

For Foucault, "only the enigma of this exteriority will remain" (1995, 290) if language finds the means of rendering everything hidden visible, of making everything serenely positive, especially in the case of madness. If neurosis were simply a constitutive form of society and no longer a deviation, then a seamless surface of language—with nothing folded, nothing hidden, everything on the outside—would be the only possible result. We have arrived at an even purer form of madness in the eradication of madness. The mad will not be like some distant horizon kept out of reach in order to define and police the norm; the mad will be folded into the norm in order to have them better disappear there.

One might wonder: is this already the possibility announced by the Freudian project? The psychoanalytic cure? Is psychoanalysis this normalization and eradication of madness? Is this the revelation of the madness of the norm? As if civilization didn't instantly produce a foreign edge but could incorporate every rupture within itself in order to do away with it finally? Is this the great therapeutic project of civilization—civilization against discontent, not civilization and its discontents? We could prophesize from the future: the very invention of psychoanalysis at the turn of the century will become the fulfillment of its wish when, only few centuries later, we find the absence of madness. Not even ordinary madness will have a face in this tranquility that history is reaching toward. "Will these traces themselves have become anything to the unknowing gaze but simply black marks?" Foucault asks with desperation (290). Why did we bother with the psychoanalysis of madness if we were always going to cancel out the edge that it occupies?

It was with palpable anxiety that Foucault wrote those lines. There is the hint of a question almost ready to vanish not only from the world in some nearby future but from his own work as well. Foucault will leave the question of literature, madness, and language behind. Collective practice replaces anything said to be merely literary or aesthetic, and madness should be folded into a question concerning a wider system and cannot be utilized in itself as anything revolutionary. Is the particularity of madness so essentially useless? Is there nothing more to do there? Are we to read this cancellation in Foucault's work as already a question about his own ambivalence toward madness and the literary and not just simply his problem with Freud?[2] While Foucault abandons the project of madness and literature, psychoanalysis in its post-Freudian offspring revives the question of psychosis, making it the cornerstone of any psychoanalytic renewal. The two seem to move in opposite directions.

To extinguish madness is to push psychiatry and psychoanalysis to their logical extremes, giving us the form of Foucault's hostility to psychoanalysis:

> So the sharp image of reason will wither in flames. The familiar game of mirroring the other side of ourselves in madness and of eavesdropping from our listening posts on voices that, coming from very far, tell us more nearly what we are—the game with its rules, its strategies, its contrivances, its tricks, its tolerated illegalities will once and for all have become nothing but a complex ritual whose significations will have been reduced to ashes.
>
> (291)

To know more nearly what we are, we listen to madness. This complex ritual, this psychoanalytic game, will have been reduced to ashes in the eradication of madness. Is this really where you think psychoanalysis was heading? That it could be this successful? Strange that Foucault says this when psychoanalysis was only beginning to define itself in relation to psychosis, to real madness as such.

Foucault says the relationship of mankind to "its ghosts," to its "bodiless pain," to its "carcass of the night" will be what is left after madness is effaced. We will render madness simply a misfortune that persists *even more* ghostly than before. If we psychoanalysts were to succeed, we would reduce the flame of an edge to ashes, destroying the space in which we might have encountered ourselves in what is truly Other. Before we have even a glimmer of a chance to think of a psychoanalysis of madness, Foucault's work razes the project.

I cannot help but hear this erasure of madness as also an erasure of the body, making the language of madness—always first bodily, concrete, literal, resistant to sense and metaphor—the only hope. What is now dying in us *is* self-estrangement, our body as parting and departing. We will only recover "the unity of the self-same" (292), an interiority with no outside. The body will be lost in this unity, while the madman tries to return the body to us by reducing language to its most literal bodily sense right as the body is about to take flight permanently.

Foucault turns this dire situation around and surprisingly says that it could be fortunate. It means, he says, that we will no longer even know how to place anything at a distance, there being no outside. Those who no longer remember how distance was created will be forced to ask: "how could humans search for their truth, for their essential speech, and their signs, in the face of a peril that made them tremble and from which they were compelled to avert their eyes once they caught sight of it?" (292). The attempt to answer a question about truth, always at a remove, without a sense of measurement to account for distance, is the purest form of Freud's statement, noted by Nancy, "Psyche is extended and knows nothing about it." Again, the Freudian project realizes itself for Foucault in shocking ways.

Impatience, Foucault says, will rear its head at the point where the future catches sight of the "same impatience with which the utterances of madness are rejected and collected, the hesitation in recognizing their emptiness and their meaningfulness" (292–93). In the future, the question "what is meaningful?" will be impossible to ask; we will be unable to decipher what is madness and what is sanity, what is true and what is false. Impatience will be a fortunate sign because, at the very least, we will have to begin all over again, searching for some radical change to self-knowledge that is no longer a catalogue of the Other's madness. There is here a psychoanalysis to come, a psychoanalysis that could take its bearing not in madness but in the traces of a disappearing madness. With madness and the body reduced to ashes, psychoanalysis could be resurrected like a phoenix.

For Foucault, looking at madness within discourse also means being able to begin to distinguish the organization that prohibition imposes within language, discerning how what is abolished internally then appears outside as a real presence (in discourse and the practices linked to it). This is an investigation that he sees as not having enough urgency. If language can be tied more closely to reality through the abolition of madness, through an eclipse of distance, language will be increasingly unhinged from sense. Language will exist more and more as a call to action, taking the form of an external practice, a means of self-ritualization. Language is not the space of reflection; it is a mode of action. Madness will be less the loop of thought than something outside. This is perhaps not a bad thing, Foucault reflects at this point, though it sounds dangerous in the ways psychosis can be.

There is something fascinating here that runs against most psychoanalytic claims. Language will be on the side of action, not reflection? Language will be on the side of external reality, not the body or subjective sense? More than this, the language of repression, the universal belief in law and taboo, does little to explain something important about the development of our relationship to discourse: "what is not allowed to appear at the level of the word, is not necessarily what is forbidden in the real of deed" (293). We can do all kinds of things that we cannot speak about. Saying and doing are split and have a varied appearance. Were we to study how what is permitted is nonetheless censored in speech, to trace what is permitted in the code but not in reality, we would only get so far. Foucault claims that "at this point, the metaphoric detour would no longer be possible, since it is the meaning itself that is the object of censorship" (294). This and that action or this and that idea are not increasingly censored; rather, meaning in itself is put under the sign of erasure. I did what I did because that's what I did. Is this development not completely terrifying?

The exclusion of madness began with sanatoriums and prisons but can now occur within any linguistic code. They don't even need the physical space of the sanatorium. This is not a world of censorship where a forbidden meaning is communicated and symbolized, like the idea of the spoken body of the hysteric communicating some desire for action. It is a more radical exclusion. It is close to what Lacan meant by foreclosure, whose simple definition can be stated as "what is abolished on the inside returns on the outside." This is close to what Foucault means by the absence of work, since what is foreclosed is not worked over by the unconscious nor preserved as a latency. There will be no more splitting of the symptom by conversion in the sense we have come to understand it.

Foucault renders the mechanism of foreclosure historical and therefore inevitable, choosing to see it as a potentially welcome change, since it is not forbidden meaning but a new position altogether:

> It says what it says, but it adds a silent surplus that quietly enunciates what it says and according to which code it says what it says. This is not the case of an encoded language but of one that is structurally esoteric. That is to say, it does not communicate a forbidden meaning by concealing its meaning; it positions itself from the start in an essential fold of the utterance.... Therefore it matters little what is said in such a language and what meaning is being delivered.
>
> (294)

What this creates for Foucault is a very "obscure" but in fact "central liberation" at the very heart of the utterance. Language becomes uncontrolled, taking flight from reality. He says, rather strikingly, "such utterance is transgressive not in its meaning, not in its verbal property, but in its *play*" (294). As meaning is foreclosed, there is a kind of liberation— you can say anything! Again, the realization of the Freudian notion of free association, speech without the imposition of meaning, is fulfilled but in a terrifying form. Foucault makes this mad psychoanalytic language of free utterance the final form of transgression and total control.

This uncontrollable flight was always a property of language, one reason that law tries to pin it down, to lock it into a set of codes or practices. For Foucault, it shows that what matters is not what is said— meaning the meaning of what is said, what is being "delivered"—but something more. This more he likens to a hollowing out, an uncontrolled silence, a surplus that is both a break with sense and its form of greatest play. Language becomes at once absolutely literal and material and, at the same time, completely unmoored from reality—madness! The attempt to remetaphorize language against this transformation is just so much psychology whose time has come.

Metaphoric speech will soon seem old, regressive, Foucault almost promises his readers. Metaphor won't even make sense to the purveyors of this new mad language, this language freed from any understanding or even reality. Freud, it seems, paved the way in both directions, shoring up an old idea of "meaningfulness" even as he recognized something new and absolutely radical in the nature of discourse, this question of loosening it from reality and the dictates of sense.

It is difficult not to sympathize with Foucault's strange attack on psychoanalysis, more serious even than Lacan's attack on psychology. Foucault admires Freud, granting him a place in this historical development that will come to wipe out his creation by fulfilling its most radical dictates:

> Freud's work ought to be taken for what it is; it does not discover that madness is apprehended in a web of significations it shares with everyday language, thereby granting the license to speak of it in the common platitudes of a psychological vocabulary.... Freud did not discover the lost identity of a meaning; he carved out the disruptive image of a signifier that is *absolutely not* like the others. This should have sufficed to shield his work from all psychologizing interpretations wherein our half of the century has buried it in the (derisive) name of the "human sciences" and their asexual union.
>
> (295)

To see this signifier that Freud found *"absolutely not"* like the others would take a more refined ear, an ear that is looking for a "central and obscure liberation ... that no culture can accept" (294). Play is the act whereby language locates not a sense in common but what is absolutely not like anything else—the jumping-off point that is the point of freedom.

The patient is on the couch babbling a mad poetics, pure play, increasingly unmoored from reality, from any demand that she be understood. This is not where an analysis begins but where it ends: it is certainly not what psychoanalysis typically means by play—this terrifying inhuman liberation. Play is the sign of the human in the human sciences, built into some silly idea about the wonders of our capacity for communication. It is not this Foucauldian unmooring from reality! Not even the obvious culprits of antipsychiatry would be able to dig us out of this psychological hole, in which, as Foucault said, they wanted us all to be buried. Take your pick—psychology or madness.

Madness creates what Foucault calls a "reserve" (akin to the hysterical preserve) that designates and exposes the place where some possibility—something yet to come—might lodge itself by sticking to this minimal point of freedom in language. Like the body of the hysteric that blocks the transmission of sense, Foucault says that we should see that Freud "exhausted its meaningless logos; he dried it out; he returned its words to their source—to that blank region of self-implication where nothing is said" (296). It also, however, might not lead to a single thing.

I find Foucault's hope here, borne by Freud, touching nevertheless. Mad language allows us to glimpse something critical unfolding and promises a site of resistance. There is a freedom in it, perhaps a new kind of freedom that makes its appearance first through the impossibility of speaking meaningfully. It holds itself in a place against the proliferation of communication, sense, rationale, and utility. In this impossibility of either speaking or being mad, madness, says Foucault, "rediscovers its sovereign right to language" (2015, 20). Madness speaks on the condition that it takes itself as an object. While this seems like an act of redoubling, folding in upon the self, in this hollow there is the possibility of a language of pure address, more pure than any neurotic language or metaphorical speech.

The twentieth century is defined by this communication that addresses no one and nothing, even or especially when claiming to do so. Then there are the mad. Mad language, on the other hand, simply asks the other to accept it, to give it the only freedom it needs to be granted, namely, the right to exist. It asks this of the other, reaching out to them without asking for translation, sense, or deciphering. It asks without demanding anything other than its own existence. "I have the impression, if I can put it this way, that very fundamentally, within us, the possibility of speaking, the possibility of being mad, are contemporaneous, and like twins, they reveal beneath our steps, the most perilous but also, possibly, the most marvelous or the most insistent of our freedoms" (25). Finally, the right to exist is equated with this narrow margin of freedom in a world that is increasingly unfree. This is the importance of the psychoanalysis of madness in a time when we have to ask: what kind of freedom are we being granted?

Foucault's touching hope is not a hope in a form of democracy or the liberal faith in human rights, sense, or correct speech, nor is it even a hope in communication or dialogue. The psychoanalysis of madness would ally itself somewhere else, putting faith in a differently inscribed freedom:

> I think we could say that, ultimately, we no longer believe in political freedom, and the dream, the famous dream of unalienated man, is now subject to ridicule. So, out of all those illusions what do we have left? Well, we have the ashes of a handful of words. And what is possible for the rest of us today, what is possible for us, we no longer entrust to things, to men, to History, to institutions, we entrust to signs.
>
> (27)

Foucault will move from this eclipse in our trust of words, of dialogue, of emancipation, to the question of writing. He says that we leave speaking behind in order to try to find in writing an evaluation of the question of a freedom that has been left in ashes. What Foucault is after here is a freedom that is not about communication, democracy, sense, meaning, or even self-reflexivity but that is a radical passage to the outside that he equates with the space of literature and the written form.

Foucault imagines a reconfiguration of space that is prefaced in the mad language of the twentieth century. Language, far from being a self-reference that allows for an interiorization in the most absolute fashion, is revealed as a merely superficial interiority. Speech and writing search for a passage to the outside. Language seeks to get as far away from itself as possible: "from the moment discourse ceases to follow the slope of self-interiorizing thought and, addressing the very being of language, returns thought to the outside, from that moment, in a single stroke, it becomes a meticulous narration of experiences, encounters, and improbable signs—language about the outside of all language, speech about the invisible side of words," writes Foucault (2006, 25). He calls this the undone form of the outside, and to place oneself there is finally to challenge the law, which, far from being something fully inside, is an outside that rules by creating an inside. It must be met *out there*, language advancing into this opening, into the outside, challenging the realm of law in order to locate freedom.

Patients have a profound sense of the futility of meaning, the failure of the institutions that were meant to provide meaning, and the extension of an interior space that leaves them receding from the world ever further, while the outside feels like being caught in a vortex of imperatives shorn of an ideal. Yet they come to a psychoanalyst. For what, we might ask? Are we not the hallmark therapy of meaning making, of inner life, precisely as an ideal? And if this is true, what does it mean to uphold an ideal? Is psychoanalysis an extension of the violence that Foucault describes? What if, following Foucault, patients come less for thoughts from the inside, for a resurrection of the empire of sense, and more out of a curiosity about the kind of clarity one can have at this extreme outer edge of oneself? What if they are coming to get outside of themselves? What if they are coming for this writing that is the only means of evaluating whatever freedom might be left to us?

The space that Foucault articulates is a space of pure transformation or conversion—as rupture and the elimination of thought, turning the world upside down or inside out, setting everything on fire in order to cross a space, to reach an edge, to touch something there and play. With a deep sense of futility, the endless loops of neurotic thought, and the erasure of the body, perhaps this mad exteriorization *is* the promise of psychoanalysis—its conversion disorder. Perhaps free association was always this exteriorization, this automaticity, this encounter with the outside. Perhaps psychoanalysis as a twentieth-century invention was, along with literature, already this means of passage, this call for an almost total departure. And the defense against psychoanalysis—against Freud's invention, the freedom of free association, and the writing of the body—is a defense against this exteriorization in an attempt to reinteriorize the subject, bring back self-reflexive language, and reestablish the smooth control of law and sense. The simple and playful right to exist is abolished in this resistance of all resistance to the madness of psychoanalysis.

IX

HOW TO SPLINTER / HOW TO BURN

Where does music go when it is not playing?—she asked herself. And disarmed she would answer: May they make a harp out of my nerves when I die.

—CLARICE LISPECTOR, *NEAR TO THE WILD HEART*

HOW TO SPLINTER

The passion of the symptom appears in a miraculous moment: when the act of signification is a moment empty of any content except itself and becomes material. It is for this reason that it is sometimes thought about as an event, the point of conversion. The analyst is there simply to mark this moment, irrespective of whether they choose to respond, to interpret. The reason for the clause is that whatever attribution of meaning might be given is negligible when it is not contraindicated. The point is to enable this moment to take place. Interpretation or silence more often clears the way here.

While this may seem like a reification or exaggeration of a process that cannot be reduced to one moment, any one point of transformation, nevertheless, if it is part of a series, should be exemplary, as should all of them taken together as a unity. The part, metonymically, can stand in for the whole. The moment of termination stands outside of this series, singular in its force as an end. But, as all psychoanalysts tend to note, the process of termination replays and contains all the moments of an analysis and is already foreshadowed by them. For reasons that are little by little coming to light, I associate the possibility that comes from this formal structure with the body.

Juliette was never told what she could be, only what she couldn't and shouldn't. The images of women in this Dominican family from the Bronx were harrowing, a fate she was consigned to and nonetheless was supposed to find a way to avoid, though without being told how. The tasks assigned to children are always so much greater than we understand. "Do not become like your devastated mother," was the superego command that sounded through the generations, consigning these women to a difficult mirror play. One has to find a means of separation from the maternal, whose sheer force of influence cannot be reduced even to the movement of identification and counteridentification. The child tries, unwittingly, to take substance from this mother and is ravaged.

Juliette often attempted a kind of recuperation through men, but men couldn't provide a point of identification in a Hispanic family where boys were still in the role of his majesty the baby and girls were consigned to the dustbin of humanity, or what we might call everything else. To watch this girl enter puberty with this injunction on her shoulders meant watching the narrow straits of conversion open up to her, the only ground available on which to map her obscure desires as a woman. I watched them take root in her body as body. So many sessions were spent on this agony in her body, the pain of being a woman, which felt to her like a curse. She tried to transfer this pain to the aesthetic care of a woman's body, which is also bound to suffering and is a variation on maternal care. These aesthetics were also colored by household war—mother-daughter fights centered on the body—a prologue to the war between the sexes.

Juliette was my very first patient. In a kind of cosmic joke, her first major symptom that erupted in the analysis was a hysterical pregnancy—a special variety of conversion disorder.[1] It's not the hysterical pregnancy itself that is of importance but the place it holds in her unfolding treatment. Juliette got her period when she was eleven, and her mother said something to her like: now you can get pregnant. It is funny writing this sentence so many years later; you can almost hear the command, the permission even—now you can. This allusion to desire is set against the prohibition—you will not—which was, at the very least, the conscious intention. This equivalence makes sense, given that women in this family only separated from their mothers by getting pregnant, by offering her a substitute in exchange for a longed-for separation.

This strange command, barely explained, had far-reaching effects on this child, who was visiting the school nurse on and off for weeks. Her mother finally called me, saying she did not know what was wrong with Juliette, could I please find out, she is complaining of stomachaches again. After a few sessions, I reconstructed the following story: there was much excitement in the home over Juliette's menstruation, and her little brother, age six, was following Juliette into the bathroom to see what all the fuss was about—no doubt a continuation of sexual games and curiosity that they had engaged in for quite some time. The whole affair was rather harmless, and up until this point, their sexual engagement with each other was probably something rather continuous, unthought, left in latency. The commandment introduced a break in this state of affairs—now you can.

Juliette's mother had strange decrees at home. For example, women's underwear was not allowed in the dirty-laundry bin and had to be washed separately. Her mother often spoke of how shameful women's bodies were, and their secretions were something that should never be seen. She reacted with panic to her daughter's body, especially her underwear, as she did her own. Her disgust did not discriminate. Juliette was constantly rushing around to hide the traces of herself, all the more pressing, one imagines, with the onset of menstruation. Again, the commandment rears its head. You cannot (leave your underwear with the rest of the family laundry) meets with her mother's you can (get pregnant), which sealed this child's fate.

Juliette's childish theory of birth was one that involved touch: things can't touch, or something bad happens. Clearly this is what pregnancy must mean, this thing that can now happen. With these little bathroom scenes where the two siblings played games around the toilet, Juliette fell into the belief that she must be pregnant, announced surreptitiously by the presence of stomachaches. If things can't touch, if her body is the site of revulsion, one thing that does touch her—as it does each of us—are words. Her body is rearranged, as happens in puberty, through these words—and everything is turned. The declarative force of these words penetrated her body—*now you can*—to which, somewhere between conversion and disorder, the body replies. Psychoanalysis is based on this premise, meaning that what has the capacity to mark is not only the site of trauma but also the agent of change.

There are two conversion symptoms in this treatment; one follows after the other. The first, stomachaches, is unraveled little by little in her analysis through telling the story of the bathroom, her talking about feeling something moving in her stomach, a sense she had that she looked bloated, and so on. Juliette finally described the moment in question: she was in the bathroom with her brother. Her little brother used the bathroom, holding his penis while he urinated, and flushed the toilet. She then used the toilet. It was touching the handle after him that was the imagined moment of conception.

I'm sure you can imagine the scene of this session, one that calls on me as her analyst to explain to her what pregnancy really is and how it happens. Touching as her story is, touching is not the reality of sex. Something about sexual difference is what is being held in abeyance. Juliette is taking up her mother's desire, a woman who didn't want to touch her daughter, especially her daughter's dirty little female body. For this little girl, she has to learn that sex is something else. Sex isn't this intrusion of a mother-daughter relationship, a maternal phobia in a complicated matrix of desire. This is something too blithely referred to in psychoanalysis as the preoedipal. This was conversion symptom number one.

After this session, a second conversion symptom emerges. Juliette has been repeatedly returning to the nurse at school, and her mother calls me. You need to speak to the girl again, and her mother brings her in for her session. What is happening this time? Juliette has a new symptom and a new fear. She said she got a splinter, and she heard that it can enter into your bloodstream and pierce your heart. A friend told this to her, and all day long she can think of nothing else. The symptom was easily interpreted. The presence of blood was not the truth about touching. It revealed another truth: not only what comes out but what can enter into her from the outside—blood comes out, a splinter can pierce one's skin and go into one's blood. Here we see the truth of her vaginal opening and, of course, the penis that may enter it. This symptom is an embodied knowledge of what was said in the previous session about sexual intercourse, and truth be told, I think it was a knowledge she already knew somewhere. All children know, according to psychoanalysis. What is fascinating is that conversion leads to a second conversion, a conversion to the second power. Conversion is not dissipated; it is intensified.

Something that only struck me many years later (I was a brand-new therapist at the time, probably too much in the role of a sex-education teacher) was the absolutely stunning character of the desire embedded in her splinter symptom. It is the desire that something may enter into her, pierce her heart, touch her. This, in a child whose mother treated her like a phobic object, by a child who was taught to fear sex. This, in a child whose model of family love was the unmitigated war between the sexes. Perhaps this was her unconscious response to an equivalence in her mother's command: now you can—this split-off permission and her split-off desire. Now you can splinter. Now you can be broken in half. Now you can separate. The symptom anticipates the moment of freedom, the moment when you finally can.

What we see here is the structuring function of symptoms—how it gives form to her desire and her body. When something splinters her, it forever changes her, like a saint whose conversion comes in a vision of being pierced in the heart by the splinters of the cross. This is her cross to bear. This is her family. This is the reality of sex. The diphasic sexual life of human beings, as Freud depicted it, is this sexuality cut in half, always bearing in it this strange splintered temporality: moments held back by latency, forced to reemerge, to return again and again. The pre-oedipal offshoots of a wild, almost anarchic sexuality force their way forward to be worked over again and again, erupting at the surface of her body.

If there is any indication of the power and passion of a conversion symptom, it is this little girl like a medieval mystic. Later in the analysis she would tell me that if she could choose a patron female religious figure, it would be the Virgin Mary, not for some hysterical disgust with sexuality but rather against that part of her heritage. She told me that the Virgin Mother is the only one who is permitted to take her body with her after death. She is also the one who is impregnated by the word, who shows us the power of words on our flesh, the consequence of which is having to bear the most brutal of maternal separations: the death of a child.

HOW TO BURN

Something crystallizes in analysis at a certain limit, and the way there isn't always paved with the analytic gold of speech and reflection. If psychoanalysis is as bodily and mad and exterior as I'm making it out to be, reaching this edge can be quite tumultuous. Analysis—the pain of it for the patient and the analyst—is too rarely spoken of. There is silence, a good deal of it, but more often there is a volatile intensity, outbreaks of symptoms, panic, changes in life that at first seem catastrophic. Indeed, one might ask the question as to why anyone would pay for more suffering. The simple answer is that some do. Some are courageous enough to pay for the cost of what it takes to make anything different, rather than simply a variation of the same.

When analysis takes off, it is true that something powerful, something uncanny, seems to be at work, which Freud likened to summoning the demons from below. But Freud cautioned his fellow analysts: "No one who, like me, conjures up the most evil of those half-tamed demons that inhabit the human breast, and seeks to wrestle with them, can expect to come through the struggle unscathed" ([1905a] 1995, 109). The analyst is the one who is scathed, burned, but the patient does not escape untouched. How do patient and analyst endure such a perilous affair—this shaking, this shock, that comes from touching what Lacan said was most opaque, most closed in one's words? The alarming thought is that I act as a dark conduit, providing a place for contingency to rear its fateful head. Whatever fantasies a patient might have of the demonic power of the analyst, this is not entirely wrong. As consolation, I remind myself that our biggest problem as psychoanalysts is that nothing happens.

Elizabeth doesn't know if she is depressed like her mother or depressed because she wants to be like her mother. They share a passion for each other, on the phone day in and day out, depression a codeword that each can mutter without having to give it any meaning really but you-and-me. The assumption that Elizabeth will share everything with her mother means that any door she closes is met with a flood of guilt. But it is hard to live with every door open. You get to keep very little of yourself.

Elizabeth came to see me after a depressive period that began after finding out about an affair her father was having. Telling the story of her relationship with her mother took her many years. They are both artisans. I write "artisans" and not "artists," for this is precisely the question; they both cannot see what they do as art. Elizabeth creates pottery from scraps, often found objects, in an elaborate ritual that plays on contingency: things find themselves together, seemingly by accident. The pieces were singular in construction, or reconstruction, and she refused to put these objects into a form of production, or reproducibility—this would detract from the contingency and singularity. Yet they were not art. She called her work her ode to waste. "How can this ever be a career?" I often wonder in some dumb parental way.

The two women shared a secret ritualistic pleasure of making for no apparent reason, though the ostensible reason was to hide from the tension of the household. The impossibility of circulation haunted them, and this closed circuit was maintained like a void they turned in together at the center of the family—a family, by the way, that included another daughter and a father. Next came the failed injunction from her mother: do not be an artist like me; put away these silly childish things. Elizabeth's craftsmanship was to become a mere hobby: she entered into the workforce, made money, received benefits, started saving. This was something her mother, as a housewife, had failed to do. Elizabeth was successful in business at a young age, though she didn't like the work much. Her life was split down the middle: she would rush home to make her pottery to finish the day with a modicum of pleasure. Her response to this split was the feeling that something was always out of joint. Pleasure was in a secret fold, while most of life was lived in the cold seamlessness of commerce and duty.

In a session, Elizabeth recalled an early symptom: she often doodled on her math tests in elementary school. Once, she even refused to take a test and found herself drawing a large sunflower across the whole page, an act her teacher took as sheer insolence. She had to bring this test home to show her parents and felt deeply ashamed; she didn't know why she had done this, so she felt childish and stupid—a feeling that would haunt the art objects she made and mercilessly devalued. This refusal to take the test seemed directed toward her mother, toward the injunction that her mother laid on her shoulders. Childish! Elizabeth's refusal was an attempt at bringing this shared shame to the surface. Like so many of the symptoms of childhood, it was not recognized as such and was simply punished. Shame meets more shame in the static enclosure of family.

One can see Elizabeth standing at a certain juncture of history, one located by Walter Benjamin around the question of the art object and its reproducibility. The original uniqueness of an art object speaks to its embeddedness in tradition, giving it an archaic, almost magical aura and a relation to ritual. The weight of an artwork's authority and authenticity is derived from tradition, which gives it durability. The technological reproducibility of art objects creates a crisis, breaking the relationship between art and religion, ritual, and magic—"a shattering of tradition which is the reverse side of the present crisis and renewal of humanity" (Benjamin 2008, 22). For the first time, reproduction emancipates the art object from its subservience to ritual at the expense of the artwork's fragile authenticity.

Certainly, this is Elizabeth's dilemma, part of the inability to choose: keep the forbidden magic at the cost of emancipation, or separate and risk losing the power of her childhood practice by entering into a thoroughly degraded adult life. This is, of course, not a choice, except perhaps the choice to figure out how to elevate this art object, a difficult task for the melancholic.

As our work together gained traction and intensity, a fateful accident happened: Elizabeth ended up with third-degree burns all over her body from a campfire mishap with a childhood friend. Physically, Elizabeth bore the brunt of injuries, and in her telling of the accident, there was almost an element of intentionality. Why might Elizabeth want to burn? The demarcating limit between me-and-you, what defines two people instead of one, is what Elizabeth and I had been speaking about in analysis. Skin is something you might think of as physically marking this limit. It was almost as if Elizabeth needed literally to *feel* this limit on her body, writing it on her skin.

Stranger still, before the accident she had an important dream where she found, to her delight, two toucans sitting on a fruit cart. The moment was memorable because I misheard her in session, and it played like an Abbott and Costello routine. "Two cans of what?" I kept asking. "No, no, not cans . . . not cans of anything, toucans, two toucans, the bird!" Even this mini *pas de deux* demonstrates the limit of two—my capacity to hear or even understand something that left the dream with a melancholic aura, now repeated in this session. In the word "toucan," we both heard "two can," which is always punctuated for her with a question mark. Two can what? It was after this dream that she asked to lie on the couch.

All of her dreams from the couch involve a magical object that one has in solitude—like the two toucans—or that, when brought into the company of others, is very difficult to access. The objects often disappear—into holes, sometimes behind walls. Once she wrote her name in the sky with fire, a self-consuming fire that wrote its own disappearance, a trace that effaced itself. This signature was done outside my office before entering. This signature in the dream followed another scene: she was in an art gallery, where she viewed something that she said looked like an abortion. Art objects in her dreams have precariousness and tend toward waste, on the verge of disappearing.

The objects she *can* have or share with another person are painfully pornographic, unsatisfying, anesthetic—the reified object of reproducibility. I think she is right in this. She identifies a necessary structural alienation. You might want to call this hysteria, the problem of *jouissance* as opposed to unfulfilled desire.[2] You would be both right and wrong. While one might be a defense against the other, dissatisfaction and complaint is a quasi-defensive way of remaining present, holding on to the contours of the object, while what disappears is truer to her felt sense of delicacy, a way of keeping herself. She is looking for something different from what can be made present or made in order to be present and then enjoyed.

Months after the accident, Elizabeth's skin had almost healed, though she was scarred. She returned to work. Life had moved on. One day, she mentioned that her mother, on a recent visit, had excitedly asked Elizabeth to recount the story of her burns and was pushing for more and more graphic detail. This made Elizabeth uncomfortable. She then told me about an episode that had previously gone unmentioned: when the hospital employees first removed her bandages to check on her wounds and the skin grafts, her mother had come into the hospital room. Ostensibly, she was there for support, but Elizabeth couldn't shake the feeling that her mother wanted to look. And here, many months later, her mother was clamoring for yet more detail.

"I said to my mother that I was really upset that she wanted me to go back to a moment that was so painful," Elizabeth told me. "And my mother replied: 'it's my trauma, too. In fact, I think I'm more traumatized by it than you.'" What were we to make of her mother's will-to-trauma, to share in trauma with her daughter? This question brought Elizabeth back to why she came to treatment in the first place: her father's affair. Elizabeth had learned of the affair because her mother had "accidentally" left a letter in plain view, which revealed the affair to her. In effect, her mother forced Elizabeth to share in the very same painful revelation, and Elizabeth felt stuck with this, forced to see it, to live with it as a trauma common to the two of them.

Elizabeth said that with the burn she finally felt that she could know something about the difference between her pain and her mother's, whereas during the letter incident she had shared in it, drowned in it even, making her mother's pain her own—as she always had. After the accident by fire, she felt that a difference had been established for the very first time. Now, you might say that this insight about her "enmeshment" with her mother was something that we could have discussed—that the burn was unnecessary to her treatment, simply coincidental. But that's precisely what I've found *isn't* the case. Even profound self-reflection seems to have very little relation to actual change. Change happens through a chance event that links to and rewrites an earlier one—an accidental letter and an accidental burn—written through her body, literally written on her skin.

After this piece of analytic work took place, I remembered an earlier scene from the toucan dream, in which she was watching something illicit on two computer screens. It had been left unanalyzed, but I had wondered during the telling of the dream about this evocation of the primal scene. It is, of course, the one we had both forgotten about—the one left in plain view by her mother. We had to rediscover the beginning of her treatment through a contingency in the treatment that erupts and reduces the maternal commandment to ashes: share my trauma, be traumatized too. We two together.

The word "case" comes from the Latin word *casus*, meaning chance event or happening. We might say that "case" means accidental event. Accidents come to life in psychoanalysis when someone is asked to speak freely, to say anything, setting off a mechanism behind the veil of speech. Freud states in his early work *Three Essays on the Theory of Sexuality*

([1905c] 1995) that when it comes to personality, the accidents of life matter most. Accidents, not heredity or biology, are destiny for Freud. Every case is a story of the accidental, where a singularity emerges from the stupor of collective narrative—the injunctions laid on one's shoulders—and returns us to a unique existence in a body, with its particular pain and its permutations of a history of joy.

If the crisis of the art object in the twenty-first century turns on reproducibility and the destruction of aura, and if the aesthetic object questions authenticity and authority, it must internalize the force of contingency, chance, accidents, giving them the level of urgency once embodied by the religious or philosophical frame. In analysis, this means breaking with collective mythology—her shared and screened traumas—to find a way that her project can sustain her. It returns something unique to the patient and draws a dividing line. Ritual need not come at the cost of bondage. The question of what two can do is addressed to me and transforms into the near-fatal encounter in the treatment— one from which she emerges with a greater sense of the weight of history, the crisis that is on her shoulders and that she cannot disinherit.

For Benjamin, renewal happens in the form of ruins, the evocation of what has been left behind, showing what is wasted in the transition to mass production. Elizabeth's relentless hymn to waste, to a writing of ashes, almost makes burning a destiny, showing that the point of renewal always comes at the cost of separation, especially from those we have loved too much. How will she make this a part of her life? What would she like to transmit differently to her children? The division in her life now actively mirrors a powerful division in life itself—between the magical object and the communal one. She knows she must invent a solution, one I know she will find in her analysis.

X

FORGED IN STONES

She sings, she who doesn't want to scream. She sings because she is proud. But one must know how to hear her. Such is her song, screamed profoundly into silence.

—HENRI MICHAUX, *LIFE IN THE FOLDS*

FORGED IN STONES

It is time to talk about the drive, a limit concept in psychoanalysis that Freud used to organize the body. Listening to the body is the same as listening to the drive circuit in an analysis—its twists and turns, these brilliant moments that flare up in dreams or in a session. This book wagers that this mode of listening to and thinking of psychoanalysis in light of conversion is also a means of rethinking the place of the psychoanalyst in this impossible profession. Let us put this wager to the test once more.

Freud talked about conversion as if it was the attempt to make stones talk, to find in the fragments or ruins of the body a map of the future. A patient often described to me an uncontrollable act of constant self-divestiture. "It is as if I have nothing at all points in time, life lived in a space of emptiness," she said. Living this way left her feeling monstrously helpless, but she seemed unwilling to stop because it constituted a particular way of being from which she nonetheless derived great pleasure. This way of living via dispossession felt to her as if she never knew what she was doing, making all encounters potentially surprising. Good. But they were also potentially horrifying. Should she arrive a little more prepared? Her answer was always unreservedly "no." When listening to her, one wishes—as an ego psychologist might—for more signal anxiety, preparation, a series of anxiety dreams, some modicum of mastery rather than this constant ravishment. Words, preparation, speech!

This lack of preparation worked well for her in her creative capacities but not, so she claimed, in a world where she is required to be self-invested rather than -divested. "Self-investiture is self-satisfaction," she exclaimed (and to hear the echo of a reaction to masturbatory *jouissance* is not wrong). "Identities," she said, "forged in stone, invested in and enjoyed, were done in the spirit of meanness." Her angry sentiment is a little too much in the register of having itself in relation to her particular ethic of disinvestment. It gives way to an identity, no less a judgment, and doesn't make its way toward the acceptance of the rejection she desperately searches for. This divestiture often throws her into her body, not out of it, indicating that she isn't in it to begin with.

One could imagine the contemporary therapist pushing her toward assertion, seeing her refusal of ownership as an inability to recognize her transgressions or failures, her inhibiting fear of exhibitionism as a morbid disposition to penis envy, a hatred of her body, or issues around self-esteem. "Why do you feel like you have nothing?" the therapist would ask smugly, or worse, "why do you choose nothing?" The therapist wouldn't necessarily be wrong, though he or she would be missing what is interesting in this patient's imperative to divest herself of every trace of identity as an attempt to be in her body. This hypothetical therapist would also miss the solutions she has found: the pleasure in secreting herself away, embodied in her writing and constitutive of it. We might recall Freud's late aphoristic remark: "Children like expressing an object relation by an identification—'I am the object.' 'Having' is the later of the two; after the loss of the object, it relapses into 'being.' Example: the breast. 'The breast is a part of me, I am the breast.' Only later: 'I have it'—that is I am not it" ([1938] 1995, 299).

The act of erasure in an amnesiac symptom attacks the links previously forged and by doing so poses the important question of what can be had. Falling back into being, this negative theology—which Lacan worries about as a slumber—leaves something radically open—too open, even. Yet it is precisely this amnesiac obfuscation, what is shut out of awareness en bloc and en masse, that makes something else possible. History lives on in this repetition, memorialized in a rhythmic liturgy to a past held in abeyance, engendered by her body, rendering the historical sonorous. She never wants to recover herself in an opening that surfaces like a gaping hole, a cry, or a howl. These sounds break the surface of her body like a wound. This pain calls on those around her—a call not limited to the psychoanalyst, though she may be in the best position to respond.

Serge Leclaire, in opposition to Jacques-Alain Miller, asked that the analyst never suture this hole, never close this opening, never offer the salvific qualities of a meaning. "The analyst," he says, "whether he likes it or not and even when he attempts to discourse upon psychoanalysis, the analyst does not suture, or at least he ought to strive to be wary of that passion" (2012, 103). He then admits that he might stop there—that statement might be the most concise form—but alas, he still must try to continue to speak of analysis. This necessity, he feels, is intolerable, almost as intolerable as it is in the face of patients.

I have learned that it would be wrong to assume that hysterical amnesia, or forgetting, isn't an act of creation. It attempts to hold open possibility in the same way repetition does. "Lord we know what we are, but not what we may be," sings Ophelia, pondering her dead father and errant lover, "may God be at your table." Contrary to Hamlet, who knows what he may be, namely, the king—but not what he is—Ophelia knows what she is. For Hamlet, the gap from nowhere to his kingly somewhere, always in the direction of an ideal, is impossible to cross. As Freud controversially commented in his 1925 paper "Some Psychical Consequences of the Anatomical Distinction Between the Sexes," the castration complex brings the Oedipus complex to grief in boys, whereas girls begin in grief. Can we not imagine with Ophelia how the leap into nothing might be taken? Is this not the reason her death in the river is represented again and again? She could have taken to it like a fish to water. Starting from the destruction of the ideal leaves an endless field of possibilities if she can avoid abjection, if she can escape getting lost in the metonymy of desire.

Melville's hysterical novel *Pierre; or, The Ambiguities* ([1852], 1996) tackles the question of love in a reenactment of Hamlet. In his final pleading lines, Pierre says:

> Here, then, is the untimely, timely end;—Life's last chapter well stitched into the middle; Nor book, nor author of the book, hath any sequel, though each hath its last lettering!—It is ambiguous still . . . I will mold a trumpet out of the flames, and, with my breath of flame, breathe back my defiance! But give me first another body! I long and long to die, to be rid of this dishonored cheek. Hung by the neck till thou be dead.—Not if I forestall you, though!—Oh now to live is death, and now to die is life; now, to my soul, were a sword my midwife!
>
> (247)

If life requires the presence of death, then life must be stitched from its middle to its end. Pierre, faced with ambiguity, can only mold a trumpet out of the flames, breathing back his defiance. But first, he asks: give me another body, a body that contains death. The midwife that Melville cries for, we might remember, is one of Freud's most important metaphors for the psychoanalyst.

But this is not a story of the birth of a subject. Poor Pierre cannot accomplish an act of rebirth or renewal, and for all his Hamlet-like contemplative philosophizing and un-Hamlet-like reconciliation of the loose threads of his past, he must stage his own death and tragic ruin. In Melville's lesson, neither contemplation nor action has the power of redemption. Any possible renewal there might be is centered on Pierre's writing of an unpublishable book, which we do not see. This manuscript functions as a kind of hidden sequel and mirror for Melville, whose published book, *Pierre; or, The Ambiguities*, was meant to be a housewife bestseller that would pull him out of bankruptcy; instead, it ends up a complete flop. Both Melville and Pierre seem to be trying to write themselves *into* ruin.

Melville did not write the book he promised his publishers, refusing the promise of monetary rebirth or financial conversion, in order to do something else, something, in the end, really quite strange: Melville merges with Pierre, dodging publishers who seek legal recourse against him. Perhaps this is a refusal inherent to hysterical amnesia, writing what cannot be written—the outcome of an important repetition. The repetition repeats the impossible, an enigmatic X, which is a baptism by flame. The amnestic strategy is a cipher that goes to the very center of being. Breathe back my defiance! Significantly, this merger between Melville and Pierre contains a book that has been written.

Same patient: When she was a little girl, like a lot of little girls, she kept a diary. One writes in a diary always a little bit hystericized. This quasi-hysterical register of writing takes place in a kind of somatic blindness where she can always claim ignorance: "I know not what I do or write." The diary plays on the border of the intimate and extimate. Its space seems wholly intimate, yet one writes for someone else's eyes, imagined and addressed . . . Dear Diary. What is inscribed on the page is felt neither to exist in the world nor in time. This patient said she never read prior entries. The space felt very close to her body. The writing was not experienced as separate from her body, this separation being one way to define existence. It was a kind of deferred separation—which I say without a trace of pathologization.

Every entry was an almost bodily appeal that solicited a new beginning. When her mother read her diary, she experienced it as the purest violation. One need only imagine the intrusion of these eyes in a space that my patient didn't even let herself know about. From that moment on, she said, everything would be written on the outside, which is how she formed herself. Not a lot can carry on hidden; she was a compulsive truth teller and gossiper and naïf whose facial expressions got her into trouble when her mouth failed to live up to its irresponsibility. "I believe," she said to me, "this started with my response to my mother's trespass—I wrote obscenities directed specifically at her on notes that I put in her closet."

It was as if I was possessed (as opposed to self-possessed). For my patient, the violation reverses course—the writing will be on the wall. So you want to see? Here! What this patient recovered in this piece of work in her analysis was a place that she could feel inviolate again in the act of writing, even when that writing was on the wall or hidden in the closet. Everything—not only diary writing—can be done as if it was never meant to be seen, even by oneself, and sometimes that is an enormous help: a little piece of repression or even, god forbid, scotomization. It is a way to hold on to wishing and a means of beginning again—putting consciousness or self-consciousness out of order, making use of the division and self-divestiture of her symptom. The fluidity of libido, Freud said, was like writing on water, opposed to the stasis of carving something into stone. Writing on water, like the work of fire, aligns with this orientation toward the object that I am, that I write myself to be.

There is a lesson here for the psychoanalyst. In a striking passage in Lacan's 1960 seminar on transference, he speaks about the forgetting of the analyst, especially as it concerns his or her position in the transference:

> The conquering of forgetting isn't quite remembering . . . it has something more to do with a mutation in the economy of the desire of the

analyst. If we really consider our relation to the unconscious we can excise that fear which we may experience of not knowing enough about ourselves. . . . I am not claiming to urge you to dispense yourselves entirely from any worry . . . but recognition of the unconscious does not in any way put the analyst beyond the reach of his passions.

(2016, 159)

Many read Freud as saying that the psychoanalytic cure aims at remembering. For Lacan, however, to conquer amnesia or repression isn't exactly a heroics of memory. It has more to do with a subjective change in libidinal economy—a mutation or conversion.

The idea of remembering as the end of analysis is essentially anal, engendering a fear that one has not learned all there is to know in order finally to do away with it, especially regarding one's irrational passions. Psychoanalysis, Lacan continues,

> is not a taming of the unconscious but rather something along the lines of the way the life drive or Eros is privileged, captivated, captured by the mainspring of the signifying chain in so far as it is what constitutes the subject of the unconscious. I would go even further—the better he is analyzed, the more it will be possible for him to be frankly in love or frankly in a state of aversion, or repulsion with regard to the most elementary modes of bodies between one another with respect to his partner.
>
> (159)

The most elementary modes of bodies—to be in a state of love or disgust, rage or aversion—are the result of psychoanalysis, not its expurgation.

One allows the drive to be captured in its unconscious elaboration; one does not use thought to block *jouissance* or the sexual drive that is articulated in the unconscious. In the grip of brutal passions, not their absence, the analyst finds his or her place:

> It is precisely in the measure that he is possessed by a desire stronger than the one that is in question, namely to get to the heart of the

matter with his patient, to take him in his arms or to throw him out the window, that happens, I would even dare say that it would augur badly for someone who never felt something like that. The analyst says, "I am possessed by a stronger desire." He is established qua analyst, in so far as there has been produced, in a word, a mutation in the economy of his desire. To conduct themselves in a game of "the loser wins."

(159)

Lacan speaks to the conversion of the patient into the analyst. This mutation in the economy of desire should not be confused with dispensing with one's unconscious, nor with knowing oneself (this horrific platitude), nor with being relieved of affective life. Rather, Lacan asks us to live with all of this at its most extreme edge and nevertheless know what it is to take up the desire of the analyst.

Be on the losing side: you do not know. The loser in this game wins. We have to lose ourselves *in* the game. It is, as I think Leclaire put it so succinctly, an intolerable desire not to suture—a hysteric's technique if there ever was one. In fact, to push the analogy with hysteria, Lacan says that it is only in knowing what desire is—having had some particular experience of it in our own analysis—but never knowing what it is for the analysand that we are finally in a position to have in ourselves this object of desire for the patient. Every manifestation of our willful having dissipates the force of the transference:

> Desire is this margin beyond the demand for the object. What the neurotic obliterates or forgets are a certain number of the most essential principles which played a part in the accidents of his access to the field of desire! ... Every premature mode of interpretation in so far as it understands too quickly ... it is in this measure that an analysis stops prematurely and in a word fails.
>
> (179)

The accidents that open the field of desire are what the neurotic forgets, as if contingency is returned to you in analysis. The economics of libidinal life change so that the patient can be stronger than a passion, even when passionately felt—especially, the passion for understanding. This is the conversion of the patient qua analyst.

FROM NOTHING TO NOTHING

The drive is a movement of repetition, and the object it snatches serves the constant renewal that cannot add up to any certain knowledge, even when there are some things we come to know or should have known better. Lacan's strange rendition of the drive is concerned with what is impossible *in* the drive—its refusal to stop or find a resting point in satisfaction—which has consequences throughout a person's life beyond mere dissatisfaction. "Even when you stuff the mouth," he writes, "it is not the food that satisfies it, it is the pleasure of the mouth. . . . Mouth comes back to the mouth" (1981, 167–68). Body returns to body even as it is exponentially extended, folded back around upon itself, exteriorized. The object, as Freud showed from the beginning, is the most indifferent aspect of this drive life.

The object is only an avatar of an always and forever lost object that sets off this bodily eruption and turning. Analysis renders the drive readable. Being more on the side of a sheer experience of movement, the drive is closer to writing than any readability, closer to movement than its capture by signification. In this way, analysis is closer to the body than to psyche, to such an extent that what an analyst does, for Lacan, in breaking speech or dismembering language, is to work on the bodily surface of language. Fundamental to this act that takes place on the level of the drive is its movement on the surface of the body, where it is felt and structured—this circular character, eternal return, repetition as formal tracing, the etching of a trajectory, and the creation of an edge. In this loop, something new will emerge, but only insofar as the loop is completed, permitted to carve its form.

"What matters is not what goes in there, as the Gospel has it, but what comes out" (144). This is the only transgression allowed in the Lacanian model—this movement toward the Other, circling the *objet a*, which is evoked as a bodily fragment. The object is lost in the field of the sexual, or lost because of it, and finally reduced to drive. Lacan says, "I suggest that there is a radical distinction between loving oneself through the other (little *a*)—which in the narcissistic field of the object, allows no transcendence to the object included—and the circularity of the drive, in which the heterogeneity of the movement out and back shows a gap in its interval" (194). The drive traverses or outlines this empty place, turns around it, and is tricked into making this turn.

Close to Freud's psyche-soma sexual schema, here Lacan's trajectory of the drive shows this puncturing of the ready-made holes in the body—the rim structure of our erogenous zones (mouth, anus, vagina, eyes, ears)—where the drive traverses another hole and makes a stitch. This

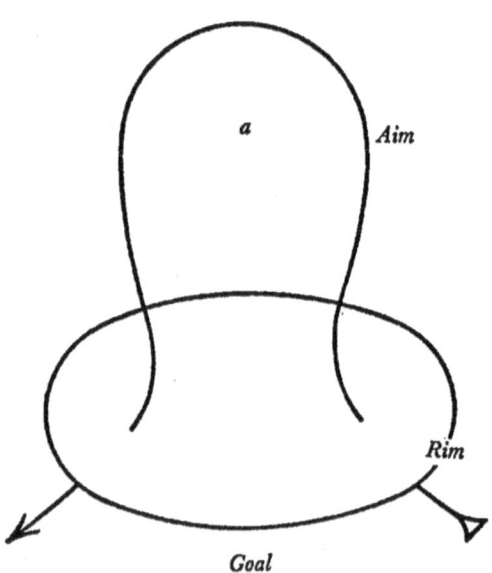

10.1 Lacan's drawing from "The Partial Drive and Its Circuit" in *Seminar XII: The Four Fundamental Concepts of Psychoanalysis.*

Source: From *The Four Fundamental Concepts of Psycho-Analysis* by Jacques Lacan, translated by Alan Sheridan, published by Chatto & Windus. Reproduced by permission of The Random House Group Ltd. © 1977.

stitch at its final point of return, might define a locus in which one might momentarily signify oneself—one way this diagram (fig. 10.1) has been read—yet it is a return into the body, which would seem antithetical to the act of self-signification. The stitch, in itself, seems to tie an original hole through a new one—from nothing to nothing, from body to body, from X back to X.

Lacan has funny ways of speaking about this movement: the blackout or syncope of the signifier, the submission to the law or castration, and the singular disappearance of the subject in the metonymy of desire. All are situated on the same level, as similar phenomena in relation to the subject's modes of disappearing, because of their body and drive. The figure of the drive obviates the repetitive movement between appearing and disappearing, the drive structured by holes on the surface of the body. The paradox of appearance in Lacan is that it is always tied to shades of disappearance. Never one without the other. Never a final act of knotting. Yet Lacan does make a distinction between this radical act of appearing and disappearing in the drive's trajectory and a narcissistic loop that cannot make this leap into the body.

Take the following dream from an analysis. *I am driving a car. My three children are in the back. I'm going too fast, and my father is across the way trying to wave at us to stop. I'm afraid. I've done something terribly wrong. My father is impotent to stop me, which I suddenly find funny because I know nothing terrible is going to happen. I can see that no other cars are coming. I slam on the brakes and skid into the intersection halfway just before I wake up.* The patient, not having crossed the gap or the intersection by putting on the brakes, wakes up feeling guilty. Nothing bad was going to happen? Why did she have to stop?

If we follow the drive, one cannot stop. What's more, stopping and repeating is different from completing the circuit and beginning again. Beginning again happens at the point when difference is achieved. In the former, nothing is transgressed—the move from nothing to nothing has not been attempted. The loop is not completed. My patient would not be subjected to the impotent law of her father, whom she derides; nor to what she knows, namely, that nothing is going to happen, really; nor even to her desire to drive off with her three children. In the last option there is a great deal of possibility. She wants to drive off—a transgressive incestuous wish—which she could satisfy in a way beyond the repetitive *agon* of fighting it out with her father (or husband) and in finding herself somewhere new. Her incestuous wish is not the same as her mother's, who in fact didn't drive off with her, much as she may have wanted to, rejecting her through a wish to merge with her symptomatically. My patient needs to complete the looping legacy of what she has inherited. With this horizon approached, the necessity to create desire anew would arise and, with it, a difference: between the generations, between satisfaction demanded and satisfaction achieved, between object lost and object present, between a lost remainder in the swell of pleasure and an excess felt in its reanimation.

The transgression by the drive into the field of the Other; the confrontation with *jouissance* in the act of circling the *objet a*; the impossibility of satisfaction, which pushes us toward the limit of difference; the necessity for repetition; and this final return to body characterize in Lacan all drives, not simply a death drive. Freud said that one never finds the death drive without Eros. They are inexorably linked, and Freud did his best to formalize a certain relationship between them that should only be taken as an ideal conceptualization. Clinical questions immediately arose in relation to the idea of a death drive but were diverted by the fascination with and fear of an aggression too intimately linked to it.

From where I stand, listening to these patients, it is not the taming of the death drive—like the neutralization of aggression or the recognition of trauma per se—that we seek as psychoanalysts. It is the removal of the blocks we erect in the face of a pleasure that only happens by virtue of the drive, especially in its deadly permutations. The rest comes of its own accord. Only when the drive is truly followed do we escape. This, again, is another way of rendering the mutation in the economy of the analyst's desire, the point of conversion.

A patient once said to me, "I can't bear opening and closing. I keep thinking this is the moment, the moment when it won't close again, that I'll have gained my ticket of admission! I have to find a way to get used to this. I close up so radically. It's like with sex, when I'm finally there I think, 'how am I not doing this all the time?' And when it's over, I can't believe what I was doing. And I forget completely the other feeling." You are always on one side of the divide or the other. Lacan said the unconscious is like a cave that, in order to gain entry, you have to knock on the door from the inside—it will never be popular with tourists, he added, in a rather serious jest. Perhaps every time we manage this knock from the inside we unite body with body, nothing with nothing, and this trace, like cave paintings on a hidden rim, are points we can return to, points where we were, in essence, knocked up.

The stitch, or quilting point, has been given short shrift lately by contemporary interpretations of psychoanalysis, interpretations linked to questions of ideology and the imaginary. It is a bad fixed point, they say. Nothing, as I'm sure you can see, seems more mobile or potentially mobile. At its very source, the drive is this movement and the rhythm of opening and closing. Patients, especially after several years of analysis, are able to begin again more quickly. Meaning always slips, and *jouissance* gnaws at the edges of a frozen edifice, rather than being a source of freezing. Using this drive potential, which is contained in the field of the sexual, is what leads to a mutation in the analyst's desire, allowing the conversion of the patient into the psychoanalyst.

In William Gaddis's first novel, *The Recognitions*, written in 1955, atonement is the name for this conversion:

> Look back, if once you're started in living, you're born into sin, then? And how do you atone? By locking yourself up in remorse for what you might have done? Or by living it through. By locking yourself up in remorse for what you know you have done? Or by going back and living it through. By locking yourself up with your work, until it becomes a gessoed surface, all prepared, clean and smooth as ivory? Or by living it through. By drawing lines in your mind? Or by living it through. If it was sin from the start, and possible all the time, to know it's possible and avoid it? . . . or to have lived it through, and live it through, and deliberately go on living it through.
>
> (1993, 896)

This atonement is a recognition, or series of recognitions rather, of what one has done. It is not a reversal or undoing of what has been done. The effects of sin cannot be avoided, nor can its cause.[1] Like movement, one has to keep going. Sin is atoned when the sinner becomes sinless not through the cessation or avoidance of sin but by owning up to what one has done and living out its consequences. It is, as it were, actively *living* one's end.

By recognizing the "end" that has been there all along, we can see the inevitability and accumulation of effects. Instead of resisting or overcoming this end, atonement resides in recognizing our role in actively creating what was paradoxically always there. Gaddis's lesson is important for the analyst and fortifies the trajectory between religion and psychoanalysis. We are decidedly not on the side of a gessoed, clean-as-ivory surface; we are not on the side of at-one-ment but of living it through atonement. Ironically, Gaddis calls this "the recognitions," which becomes the title of his novel.

PULL YOU DOWN

Lacan elevates and universalizes hysteria and hysterical amnesia as constitutive of the subject, the ultimate conversion. The psychoanalytic cure aims not for restoration but for the callous grace of this headless, diary-writing, self-divested voice that knows not what it does. This self-eclipse is wed to the *mise en abyme* of the unconscious. Lacan pushes hysteria into the abyss so we might find out how better to live there.

For Lacan, the abyss is the locus of apocalyptic desire or *jouissance*. Why is satisfaction apocalyptic? The hysteric's desire is a desire for an unsatisfied desire—we know the mantra. But clinically, the hysteric is a question concerning how each patient can live by keeping satisfaction in abeyance and how this abeyance forms the center, the crux, of an unfolding treatment as it makes its way toward what was staved off or starved, like the butcher's wife's friend she dreamed of not wanting to feed. The center here is not on the side of meaning. It is a body event, this starvation and the series of objects that are called forth from the depths.

Lacan criticizes the psychoanalyst's hoisting up the symptom, through which the hysteric satisfies herself unbeknownst to herself, as the truth. It doesn't mean that there isn't truth, certainly there is, but it is not simply the restoration of meaning that is her cure. Her cure is on the side of a confrontation with her body, and this confrontation is always apocalyptic. It shreds the last vestiges of self, pushing her toward the utmost limit, positioning her there where she is not, in the hole of her own forgetting, facing the writing on the wall.

After forcing a seventeen-year-old patient of mine to write down his dreams three years into treatment, after he toyed with me in session about having dreams but forgetting them, he had the following dream: *I am in an old medical room, you know, like the ones you see in the pictures that they use for teaching, like they are round and there are bleachers where people watch. You know what I'm talking about. Yes? Well, it's there, and I can't see who is in the audience, all blurry anonymous faces, and I'm on an operating table, and you are carving me like a turkey. Just removing huge chunks of me and putting them in a bucket, and I don't want you to know how much it hurts. You were just going at it.*

After much discussion of the dream—a dream he more or less interpreted himself with ease—I asked him if I was going at it because I didn't know that it hurt him. He had said that in the dream he hid his pain very well. He replied that he didn't know if that is why I was going at it but asked me very directly, "now that you do know, will you do anything differently?" I looked at him quizzically. "Probably not," he said, "you're so goddamn evil . . . that look on your face . . . but this was a lot of fun, more fun than I thought." The dream had a profound impact on me.

First of all, it was funny when he was telling it to me, playing at accusing me of being a total sadist. Violence and humor mix with rapid force, a sardonic attack that stretches in both directions. More poignantly, this young boy reimagined the primal scene of psychoanalysis: Charcot with the hysterics at the Salpêtrière, adding the element of cutting so important to Lacan. The analyst has probably always been a demonic Faustian figure who demands a pound of flesh, the one whose desire is imagined to be something brutal. His appeal to me not to do anything differently in the face of his pain is certainly a desire he holds for himself, a wish to sustain his desire, even if that necessitates a kind of cruelty—namely, the brutality of drive, pure and simple.

Jouissance marks this transgressive violence. This dream was certainly a first link to the drive, and it is also a response to having displayed my desire as analyst, forcing him to bring me dreams. The weirdness of the analytic relationship is contained in the dream image—amphitheater turkey carving, translating the untranslatable act of talking about dreams and the body. Is the comedic undertone, its place in the transference, what allows this dream not to be a nightmare? Does the violent comedy of analysis spell the possibility of something new in his life, something like sublimation and the road toward it? Or is it simply defense?

He had another dream: "I jack a car, pulling the driver from the driver's seat, get in, drive it recklessly, crash it, get out, and do it again. I jack another car, pull the driver out, drive it around the block, crash it, do it again . . . and then, guess what?" He looks at me. "What?" I respond. He makes a well-timed, comedic pause. "Well," he continues, "I jack another car, pull the driver to the ground, get in, drive it around the block, crash it, I jack another car, pull the driver to the ground, get in, drive it around the block, crash it, and I do it again. And again, and again." There was a joke in the dream about repetition—repetition itself a pivot between humor and its other side, brute tragedy. He allows this other side and his fear to creep in: it felt like it went on forever; it felt like it would never stop.

Lacan told the dream of one of his patients at a conference in Leuven in 1969.[2] She dreamed of infinite lives springing from her in succession, a Pascalian dream of being engulfed in an infinity from which she awoke half-mad. As the audience burst into laughter, he assured them that while it might seem funny, it was not, in the slightest, funny to her. Infinite repetition is madness incarnate, and there is a madness in this dream of carjacking. But the infinity points the way forward. The "endless, pointless, chaotic, violence," as he put it, was a metaphor for his tie to his mother—a maddening masturbatory jacking-off game they both shared and that neither could end. "It ends when I pull her down with me," he told me in a state of glee. "I'm in this fight to the death. I've got it all mapped out." And he did, it is true. He had told me the rules of the game for the past year. I painfully lived through it with them.

The *jouissance* in this dream was even more palpable than the first. There in the sexual language—pull her down with me—but also in the rhythm of the dream, pulling one off again and again and again. "And you spare me such torture?" I asked him at one point. "I don't think I can win against you," he quipped. This is not entirely true, since some game of withholding was certainly at play, an obsessional strategy I took on by force, forcing him to tell me his dreams. It is not a tactic I generally use, but something moved me to try to break up a kind of dead repetition. One lives through games, games that my patient managed to force (with difficulty) into the intersubjective arena. I did him the service of likewise forcing some of this into the arena of his psychoanalysis.

From my perspective, his satisfaction was never totally insular, although it could become so during his early periodic depressions and for periods in the analysis. Three years into treatment, he could exude a new charm in his life, in particular when he "played games" with his friends, with authority, and with girls. The game is something he loves constantly to renew in an upping of the stakes, which he relishes. He taunts me in every session: Let's make a bet! While he attributes, in the dream, the demonic force to me—someone he sees as asking him to play every session—it is he who has set the frame. Every session feels like a renewal of a command. What are you going to talk about today? How far will we take this? This is how I would describe the particular exigency of the question that emerges in his analysis: in what way can we play with an elusive pleasure, always bordering on sadism, so that we aren't just engaged in pointless repetition?

After the carjacking dream, I pointed out to him that he wanted his own car, that for the first time he would be in the driver's seat if he got one, and that most of the fights with his mother took place with him in the passenger seat, especially when she drove him to see me. "I'm going to car jack that bitch, pull her out of the driver's seat," he squealed with delight. He then told me that the car he picked out was the same car his father drove when he was young. A Datsun. He didn't remember that. His mother told him. I don't doubt that the "Da" joined to the "son" in the name of the car is not coincidental. But then again, I wouldn't.

Is it always this iteration of an Oedipal story that is the force behind repetition—violent, incestuously sexual, hilarious? Does masturbatory *jouissance* always rear its head in the Oedipal joke? Sheer symptomatic repetition in treatments, as many of us know, feels lethal, and we perk up as the work of analysis mutates this repetition into something else. But the something else, at least as I'm thinking of it with this patient, is still repetition.

Lacan's distinction between the repetition of a need and the need for repetition is crucial. He locates the first as a collapse of desire into interminable need and frustration, landing one in a stuck economy, hankering after objects that tend more toward a zero than the tension of iteration and the play of difference. The second—the need for repetition—is located at the boundary between the symbolic and the real, the place where language brings itself to bear on one's life, forcing us into an interminable search for what is already accepted as lost, to take up this circuit of the drive. As Serge Leclaire described it:

> The driving factor is the difference between the pleasure demanded and that which is achieved. It is this difference that is expressed in the drives but also in the signifiers that emerge from their repression. The drive therefore appears as the dynamic of difference, and it would be justified to say that the goal of the drive is to maintain this difference, because by virtue of the satisfaction it demands, it re-animates at every instance the experience of a difference with the memory of primary satisfaction.
>
> (1966, 133)

What Leclaire is showing here is how drive is structured through repetition, but repetition is always accompanied by difference. If we search time and again for the same lost object, turning around this hole, we nonetheless find ourselves somewhere new and unexpected. The drive needs the force of repetition—transgressive, on the edge of violence, often flying in the face of reality—with which it carves this trajectory in the world, writes it on the surface of the body. But it is not the aim in the end (always the lost object) but the way taken, this writing, that is of importance.

Heidegger (1971) makes an important distinction between the repetition of tradition and the repetition of heritage. Tradition is the repetition of something dead and sedimented; heritage is a reactivated tradition submitted to what Heidegger calls *Wiederholung*, which can be translated as both "repetition" and "fetching back." Paradoxically, the condition for newness in Heidegger is the repetition of repetition, a kind of second-order repetition of greater intensity. Not, I would say, the bitching in the car that happened over and over and over but the wild exclamation: *Carjack that bitch!* This reminds me of Lacan's command, taken from Revelations, to "eat the book." This command joins up with Lacan's ethical injunction: live in conformity with the desire that is in you. Indeed, the two—eating the book and raising the object to the dignity of the thing—form the play of his characterization of the ethics of psychoanalysis.

Having linked desire to the lost object, what Lacan points to is a kind of faith that follows the drive. Like the potter who sculpts his vase around an interior emptiness, what is made is made there in the work of repetition. Like infinite carjacking, with its acknowledged horizon of *jouissance*. *Jouissance* contains history, a history that is fetched back, relived, repeated, if not sublimated. One of my patient's main symptoms was kleptomania. The car he doesn't know that he infinitely steals, drives, and crashes is his father's; it is his means of separation from his mother. Far from renouncing his wish, the analysis brings about its demonic fulfillment.

NO PLACE FOR THE PSYCHOANALYST

To end, I would like to return to Serge Leclaire's impossible call for an unsutured desire, a desire that leaves the analyst asking: what and how can I write or speak about psychoanalysis? Recently, it was revealed to me that there has been some suspicion regarding Leclaire's infamous patient who dreams of the unicorn (1998), that it was not a patient but actually Leclaire. The analysis, then, would be his own self-analysis. How is this possible? I was shocked by this potential revelation, angry even—the liar! He and Kohut, arm in arm, the French and American analysts obsessed with primary narcissism—they both wrote falsified treatments that were their own!

On further reflection, it occurred to me that the rage stemmed from my own countertransference, because Leclaire's analysis of the man who dreamed of the unicorn formed part of a menacing professional superego—if real analysis looks like this, then what the hell am I doing? Knowing this, it occurred to me that only from self-analysis can we glean the miraculous unfolding details exemplified in this case, something you see only at the end of an analysis. Something else happened in analysis proper—this change in the economy of desire that Lacan signals. But the minimal difference between that change in libidinal economy and what takes place in his writing was, and is, an incredibly important distinction for me.

One can work on these details regarding the signifiers in one's life but only after the libidinal conversion has taken place, leading to the conversion of the patient into the psychoanalyst. This is the moment when the circuit of the drive is completed, at least once, most likely several times over, which leads to the termination phase. Freud, for example, could only examine his dreams after his transferential exchange with Fliess. Lineaments of the work are there during analysis, but it is not, and never will be, anything total or full. There is no grand unfolding of the case.

Leclaire's writing is a wonderful afterimage. Something about what is possible postanalysis—part of self-analysis, as it is too blithely called. I had to encounter this difference in him before I understood what kind of play psychoanalysis enables. This failure, this ignorance even, to make the distinction reminds me of the deadliness of ideals, the destructiveness of imagining too quickly the end of any analysis. What encounter remains? I would like to name this residue *the* imaginary of psychoanalysis. What is there when the analyst declares with righteousness: this is not psychoanalysis! Or worse: this *is* psychoanalysis!

What has been important for me in Leclaire's work is always his reference to the true object of analysis: the drive and the unknown achievement that can be gained in following its movement and modes of appearance as rigorously as possible. This, he promises, will always bring to the surface something absolutely crucial to the patient and his or her cure. He makes this promise but never says anything about how it *should* look. It's a rather hearty declaration, while the discourse as discourse is rather thin. But I think Leclaire wants it this way, and his words could be soothing.

In the end, Leclaire reveals himself not as a speaker or even a theoretician but as a listener. The analyst listens to discourse and then must confront the task of writing something equal to this listening. He never lets on that this will be easy—quite to the contrary: "The domain of the analyst is a domain that is necessarily a-veridical, at least in its exercise . . . in fact, he does not construct a discourse, even when he speaks . . . the analyst . . . is more like the subject of the unconscious, which is to say that he has no place and cannot have one. . . . Only one thing is sure: the day the analyst is in his place, there will no longer be analysis" (2006, 105–6). There can be no place for the psychoanalyst who constructs a discourse. The irony is that despite knowing this, I sutured Leclaire. I used him to put the analyst in her place, forming an impossible ideal. In what I am writing now, in this treatise on hysteria and conversion disorder, I am trying to displace the analyst. This impossible-to-write book about the body is certainly about the impossible position of the psychoanalyst.

XI

THE SLIDING OF THE RING

It remains to make an appeal to where the affair takes place. And it can only be in the structure that the psychoanalyst shows as a symptom, when suddenly struck by an inverted Grace, he comes to raise an idolatrous prayer to "his ear," a fetish that has arisen in his breast along a hypochondriacal path. There is an area of stigmata that living in this field imposes, because of failing to map out the sense of the psychoanalytic act. It presents itself rather painfully in the penumbra of councils which the collectivity identified by it, takes on the image of a parodied church.

—JACQUES LACAN, *THE PSYCHOANALYTIC ACT*

THE SLIDING OF THE RING

In his short paper from 1935 entitled "The Subtleties of a Faulty Action," it is as if Freud needed to remind us that faulty action is not necessarily obvious or robust but subtle. By implication, there is a relationship between fallaciousness and subtlety, mistakes that travel undercover, hidden, waiting. Hiding in plain sight usually invokes the presence of death in Freud. And in this little paper, the question of subtlety is a reminder to the analyst that all self-analysis is incomplete, that our judgments of value follow our wish for happiness, that our actions often fail or symptomatically short-circuit, and that finally none of us wants to look death clearly in the face. Maybe the subtlety of a faulty action will call us to order. Maybe it will remind us that the conversion experience of psychoanalysis is not a one-time affair, a virginity lost, but something we must find a way to do, again and again. Perhaps this repetition, this persistence, is something we can endure with a little more ease, take on as simply a condition of living, especially living with others. Perhaps it ceases to be such a burden or fault?

This paper is a strange cautionary tale written late in the game, a lesson that at face value seems rather commonplace—namely, the analyzability of a parapraxis, something Freud certainly established early on, in 1901, in *The Psychopathology of Everyday Life*. The short paper, two pages at most, was written in 1935, just before the much more famous "A Disturbance of Memory on the Acropolis." Freud moves from faulty symptomatic action to disturbances of memory and time; one seems to focus on women and daughters, the other on fathers and brothers. In the paper on faulty action, the mistake that takes center stage is a slip of the pen, a mistake when writing out instructions for a gift, the smallest of mistakes, but concealing a "large number of premises and dynamic determinants" ([1935] 1995, 235). Small mistakes, large motives. It would probably do us some good to remember that a fault is not only a mistake but also an opening, a crevice into which one might fall. In this little self-study, Freud even seems to insinuate that the mistake isn't a mistake. It is the attempt at a mistake, a word that is written and crossed out immediately, a mistake that autocorrected another mistake, a stylistic repetition that the mistaken word alerted Freud to. This is the subtlety. But it is precisely here that this paper folds in on itself.

Freud accidentally writes the word *bis*—which means "till" or "until" in German and "for a second time" in Latin—at a point in which he writes *für*, or "for," twice, "in rapid succession." This repetition of *for* "sounded ugly and should be avoided" (233). The phonetic equivocal meaning in two languages of *bis*, *until*, and *for a second time* links with the German *für* and substitutes for it. Freud is alerted to the repetition of *for* by the internal repetition inherent to *bis*, which he remembers in the Latin expression "*ne bis in idem*," "do not institute the same proceedings twice," a maxim of Roman law. Or, "bis! bis!" in French, when Frenchmen cry for a repeat performance, an encore. The action thus stretches between giving, for, until, for a second time, again, never again, not twice, and the paradoxical maxim "do not create an institution from this repetition."

The immediacy of action in the giving of a gift is interrupted by a slight mistake, which introduces a delay—*until*—and then a question, *more or never again*? The mistake achieves significance not in being made but in being corrected. The repetition is done away with, or undone. This structure is explicit, he says, in many parapraxes. The faulty action, then, is not an action at all but an undoing of action, an action that points to its undoing, and this doing and undoing is the force of repetition. What is fascinating is that Freud says he would have been satisfied with this aesthetic explanation, the removal of the rather ugly repetition of *for*, except that one needs to avoid the danger of incomplete interpretation when it comes to self-analysis. We should not be satisfied too quickly. There is more. *Bis*!

Freud turns the example over to his daughter, Anna Freud, who reminded him that he had given that same gift to the same woman already. The woman happened to be Dorothy Burlingham, and this repeated gift to her was most likely the repetition he wanted to avoid. It isn't nice to give the same gift twice. Behind the repetition of the word and the wrong word for the right action we find yet another repetition—this time in reality—of the gift: the same ring with an engraved gem. Why does Freud want to give this gift twice?

In fact, it seems that he didn't *not* want to give the gift again as an act of impropriety but rather that, in the first place, he never wanted to give it at all. "For it is easy to discover the further sequel. I was looking for a motive for not making a present of the stone, and that motive was provided by the reflection that I had already made the same (or a very similar) present. Why should this object have been concealed or disguised? Very soon I saw clearly why. I wanted not to give the stone away at all. I liked it very much myself" (234). In giving the gift twice, he would have created a motive not to give the gift to Dorothy Burlingham but to himself. Freud consoles himself with the thought that "regrets of this kind only enhance the value of the gift. What sort of gift would it be if one were not a little bit sorry to part with it?" (234). This raises the gift to a second power: Freud is not just giving it twice but potentially losing it twice. It functions as both this double loss while also being yet another renunciation of the act of giving, a reassertion of selfishness.

Really to give something one must experience the gift as a loss, and it is precisely this loss that makes its appearance in the repetition, in the space between again and never again. An intense ambivalence appears, and it isn't clear whether the never again—the figure of death contained in the loss—is what he is trying to prevent or trying to encounter. Losing it twice, it is an action that is not simply an undoing of a prior action but an action intensified through repetition. Even further, he brings in his daughter—implicated in the gift—supposedly to check that his analysis is sound, moving even closer to action, to the completion of the repetition.

Why did Freud write this short text in 1935? Nothing methodologically new makes an appearance; the discovery seems rather old. Perhaps we ought to link this paper to his next, "A Disturbance of Memory on the Acropolis" ([1936] 1995), where there is an affective play between having gone too far, the experience of unreality, and filial piety. Freud, visiting the Acropolis with his brother, interprets his disbelief as a disturbance of memory, a tear in the fabric of reality that happens on the basis of confronting a moment of surpassing his own father, who was too poor to travel. "So it exists!" is a translation of "I never thought I would make it this far" or "this is too good to be true." Freud is talking about the unreality that comes from crossing a certain line, from fulfilling a long-held wish.

Guilt appears in this doubling of consciousness—this is and is not happening—which evokes a certain low mood. Even further, the disavowed satisfaction can serve as a strong motive to fall ill, which is opposed to the general rule of neurotic illness as a result of frustration. This reversal in the symptom, Freud says, is the intergenerational transmission of guilt through the superego—the death drive passed down—haunting those who are wrecked by success. The limit is set; the law is laid down; transgression is a punishable offence. One is commanded: do not go further than where I am.

A question remains: did Freud go too far, or did he not go far enough? There is something about the failed gift, the half-gift, the reluctant gift, in this paternal exchange. Is the gift of life a gift at all when half-given? The gift soon becomes a curse, something Lacan called the *me phynai* of Oedipus—better not to have been born. This is a sort of half-action in life; a half-complete circuit causes life to slip from being to nonbeing and back, made apparent in any feeling of derealization. Does it exist? Do I exist? Nonbeing appears in every slip, every disturbance, and every satisfaction; it demands a profound confrontation, like that on the Acropolis. Freud's refusal to give the ring, by giving it twice, signals his own ambivalence, not in some silly psychodrama about his daughter, whom he didn't want to renounce to her lover— though there is that—but more as a warning to himself.

Perhaps at this point we should evoke in our own analysis the fate of Freud's secret committee and the seven rings given to his anointed seven sons (see Grosskurth 1991), now repeated later in life with the women who surrounded him, including his daughter Anna and her secret lover, Dorothy Burlingham. Of course, in this death-driven exchange of gifts, one cannot help but think of Freud's 1913 paper "The Theme of the Three Caskets," where the demand for filial piety is the ruin of King Lear and the destruction of his kingdom, causing the death of his beloved daughter, Cordelia, who refuses to provide proof of her love for her father in exchange for a portion of his wealth. In the logic of forced choice, Freud shows that to choose love is always to choose death: "King Lear's dramatic story is intended to inculcate two wise lessons: that one should not give up one's possessions and rights during one's lifetime, and that one must guard against accepting flattery at its face value" ([1913a] 1995, 300). Father, can't you see?

Oddly enough, this is a mistake both Freud and Lacan make: anointing heirs and playing a game of loyalty to the Father. "Analysis Terminable and Interminable," written by Freud in 1937, is foreshadowed in the paper on "a faulty action," which can be read as a warning to future analysts against incomplete analysis. Hidden in plain sight, this rarely discussed paper becomes a critical reference point. If Freud claims that there is a bedrock refusal of castration or death, then is analysis unending? If an obstinate desire for mastery is equally present in both sexes, where illness is preferable to cure, then is analysis unending? Freud says the most difficult point is when the patient must recognize the help coming from the other, a recognition of the analyst's gift, meaning one didn't have it to begin with. It is here that most analyses break down.

So how can analysis end? Or is it unending because—to the very end—our motives will always be hidden, because we will always revert to this baseline refusal of a gift? The problem that Freud is outlining in 1937 concerns the "negative therapeutic reaction," or the negative side of transference—hate, not love, or ambivalence more generally. The patient wants to remain ill to show his hate rather than get well as a result of his love. This conundrum was first signaled in the 1920s, when the early successes of psychoanalytic treatment seemed to disappear. The insights had grown too commonplace, or insight, in the way it was conceived at that time, wasn't proving any longer to be the operative force of treatment, causing Freud to rewrite the economics of the libido. We do not simply seek pleasure: we go beyond the pleasure principle—a beyond where what is pleasure and what is unpleasure, what is life and what is death, what is love and what is hate, what is a gift and what is not, are much more difficult to distinguish.

The relentlessness of this beyond is why analysts may need to return, again and again, for analysis, like maintenance or a hygienic practice.

Even Freud, who was never analyzed, said this! The libidinal rewrite post-1920 suggests that there must be a more radical structural shift beyond insight into unconscious motivations. The beyond of the pleasure principle is the problem of the more and more, which must be the basis for some kind of encounter in an analysis. Is there any more significant encounter with the unconscious that can bring the analysis to an end? Is there a change in the libidinal economy pointed to by the term "sublimation," where pleasure remains intact and bypasses repression? Is there a decisive conversion? For Lacan, the analyst must be possessed by this more and more, this monstrousness of the drive in the form of the desire of the analyst, something that he also calls the ethics of psychoanalysis (1997). A strange reversal, but that's Lacan for you.

Sublimation outlines a point where the ego-ideal and the capacity to produce something that provides satisfaction (in contrast to those wrecked by success, the guilty, and the self-punitive) converge, rather than falling prey to the neurotic system that moves them further and further apart. For Lacan, the analyst must be possessed by a desire that goes beyond the cheaper or more illusory satisfactions offered. We might name this the conversion of the psychoanalyst. While Freud ruthlessly devoured his sons, whom he saw as either loyal and subservient or rebellious and heretical, Lacan (at least in his self-presentation) seems to invert this infanticidal process, feeling himself devoured by the ruthlessness of his psychoanalytic parent institution and asking his followers to refuse him. Lacan desired a sublimation-oriented psychoanalytic institution where the transformation required in analysis—the conversion of the analyst—would be mirrored in the profession and in the professional body.

If, for Freud, love was always an illusion that would eventually betray one's ambivalence and death wish toward loved ones, Lacan was someone for whom death could become the gift of love, the giving and receiving of nothing. Love is an intersubjective game of recognition that plays with the loss at the heart of loving. At its extreme end, love is an act of submission, an acceptance of powerlessness in the face of the other, ceding something of oneself to them. While this might look like dominance and submission, both parties in the end cede to what is beyond either of them, showing that what is neither mine nor yours is potentially ours, insofar as it will never be ours to have. Is this not the very paradoxical definition of what a psychoanalytic institution must be? A group of people centered on a love of the unconscious?

Lacan's definition of love thus tries to account for Freud's beyond by bringing in both wish and wound, old and new, in the ever-present fault and faulty actions of loving partners. He says that it was precisely this double movement in Freud that affected him deeply. It is where he began with psychoanalysis:

> The beginning of wisdom should involve beginning to realize that it is in that respect that old father Freud broke new ground. I myself began with that because it affected me quite a bit. It could affect anyone, moreover, couldn't it, to realize that love, while it is true that it has a relationship with the One, never makes anyone leave himself behind.... How can there be love for another?
>
> (1999, 47)

In this Lacanian vein, Freud's love tokens, the death rings, may signify the recognition of frailty and fault rather than its refusal. The ring is not a symbol of the One, the unity of Freud and his followers in a parodic church, but the gift of an enclosed hole, the hole transferred from analyst to analyst. The mistaken writing of *bis*, bringing in his daughter Anna to analyze him, reversing their roles, asks the other to go on, to continue, to undo the repetition of *for* through an act of hyper-repetition. A repetition that tries to go beyond, to exhaust itself, to meet its end, and only then to confer something of value and accept the exchange: my loss, your gain.

But perhaps this is mere wishful thinking on my part. Especially since, on further reflection, the Lacanian institution is as tragicomic as Freud's, marked also by the *me phynai*, better that it was not born. The anointing of the favorite son, the creation of another worldwide institution, the hierarchy of designated analysts, is all too repetitious. One seems not to have gone beyond the other much, if at all. Love never made anyone leave themselves behind, as Lacan tells us. To Freud's *bis* we can add Lacan's *encore*—two psychoanalysts and their call for more and more, directed at their children: prove to me your love.

Lacan ends the seminar in 1972–1973 that bears the name *Encore* with this strangely triumphant exultation to his followers:

> There—I'm leaving you.
>
> Shall I say, "See you next year"? You'll notice I've never ever said that to you. For a very simple reason—which is that I've never known, for the last twenty years, if I would continue next year.... Why not stop the encore now?
>
> (1998, 146)

As always, Lacan ends his seminar abruptly, with a thousand loose ends. But this time he marks the end—I'm leaving you—contextualizing this moment as one that has gone on for twenty years. He's never known if he would come back. The question of stopping has been there every time he's said goodbye. He continues: "What is truly admirable is that no one ever doubted that I would continue. The fact that I am making this remark nevertheless raises the question. It could, after all, happen that to the encore I add—'That's enough'" (146). He seems to taunt the audience, saying it is admirable that they never doubted he would continue, imagining that he would be there year after year. But why? Couldn't they imagine that he would at some point have had enough of it? That even when you say "again," the end is always possible?

Lacan is playing here with the question of the end of analysis, an end that is present in the ending of every session. The patient needs to believe that the analyst will always be there, will never leave, but should this admirable illusion be allowed to remain:

> Well, I'll leave it for you to place your bets on. There are many who believe they know me and who think I find herein an infinite satisfaction. Next to the amount of work it involves, I must say that that seems pretty minimal to me. So place your bets.

> And what will the results be? Will it mean that those who have guessed correctly love me? Well . . . to know what your partner will do is not a proof of love.
>
> (146)

It's an obscure and contradictory ending to a seminar where Lacan seems consistently to push against his audience, claiming that he doesn't want to know anything about what he teaches, that he's amazed he's still (*encore*) there and that they are too. He would like them to leave or, at least, for their numbers to drop. Their leaving—rather than assuming that he will infinitely stay and that they will be infinitely satisfied by his teaching—could reveal an important sign of protest. Only then could he imagine they were actually listening to him.

I'm leaving . . . a proof of love does not mean knowing what I will do—Lacan taunts the audience members, who imagine that his showing up again and again means that he loves them. The audience seems unable to reach the point *he* is at, or, as he says, "they still have a way to go." Only when what they have seems adequate to them, adequate enough at least to speak, to stop looking to him for it—will they detach themselves. Separate! This is presumably supposed to happen in psychoanalysis, he says. I ask you to refuse what I offer to you because that's not it. Lacan can ask this of his audience because the place from which he speaks, he declares counterintuitively, is from the position of the analysand. He carries on talking like a patient. There cannot be an infinite satisfaction derived from listening to this talking. There must be a moment when an *enough* appears!

Yet Lacan doesn't decide that he has had *enough*—a job better suited for an analysand than the analyst, who, ostensibly, isn't allowed to quit, even if they are allowed to bring sessions to an end, sometimes when they want. From which position does Lacan ask the other to leave—analyst or analysand? He keeps talking, asking the audience why *they* don't leave him, something common enough in clinical work: why do you sit there listening to me, why do you let me come here, why don't you tell me just to leave or leave yourself? A series of demands addressed to one's analyst that evade the fact that one has asked the analyst to come and is paying to do so.

It's a negative declaration of love: asking the other to ask them to stay, interrogating the other's love. While Lacan seems to want proof of the audience's capacity to absent themselves, perhaps we should read in this a double desire for the fall of the analyst implicit in the demand for love. Like the object of anxiety, we want to survive the fall, not strive for permanence or even some imagined perfect attachment. Lacan will continue his seminar for another seven years after *Encore*, carrying on with this audience, who could do better than loving him as the analyst, the subject supposed to know, by finding themselves in the position of analyst to Lacan.

Lacan starts a session of *Encore* with something rare for him, a dream of his own, saying, "I dreamt last night that when I arrived no one was here." He goes on: "That confirms the wishful character of the dream. Despite the fact that I was rather outraged, that it would all be for naught, since I also remembered in the dream that I had worked until 4:30 in the morning, it was nevertheless the satisfaction of a wish, namely, that then I would have but to twiddle my thumbs" (118). While he says that he would like to twiddle his thumbs alone, Lacan is also upset that it might be "all for naught," in this rather typical anxiety dream. He is at pains to remind himself that he had worked till 4:30 in the morning, signaling an intrusion of consciousness and reality into the dream text. He holds to this reality against the wish of the dream—either that everyone is there or no one is. No matter which direction the desire goes, his need for his audience is palpable, even if he is trying to master this need by dreaming them away.

There is a problem in Lacan's gesture of asking the audience that he calls on to disappear, especially when he states that what keeps him there—the satisfaction he is after—is to be able to please himself or get angry and feel abandoned. Probably, they are ambivalently the same thing. But another, altogether different possibility remains: to dream of his own disappearance, to realize the anxiety of "all for naught," and in so doing open in this audience a listening analytic ear. The audience has not gone missing—this strange demand. Lacan goes missing. Enough! I'm really leaving you this time.

Lacan attributes to Gide the same desire to disappear in his text "The Youth of Gide, or, The Letter of Desire," in which he claims Gide wrote letters in order for them to be burned by his wife:

> Hence Gide's groan—that of a female primate struck in the stomach, wailing over the ripping away of these letters that were a doubling of himself, which is why he calls them his child—can but seem precisely to fill the very gap that the woman's act wished to open up in his being, deepening it slowly as one after the other of the letters was thrown onto the fire of his blazing soul.
>
> (2006, 640)

Gide's courage in the end, Lacan declared, "failed him"—the burned letters represented the withdrawal of his desire, his inability to support this disappearance, and thus the end of his writing. The Marquis de Sade, on the other hand, goes all the way. Lacan claims that far from Sade's desire as author being governed by a sadistic fantasy, or even showing himself as the other face of moral law, Sade's desire was a desire to disappear, for "as a subject it is through his disappearance that he makes his mark" (657). His image is eclipsed; his extraordinary writing remains. Marguerite Duras, whom Lacan praises for understanding the essence of feminine madness, is likewise said to show us how "in Love's guessing game you lose yourself" (1987, 122).

Knowing will never prove anything. This is the limit Lacan wants the analysand to encounter. It is part of the reason for his variations on the standard form of psychoanalytic treatment (varying the four- or-five-times-a-week, forty-five or fifty-minute session, with minimal interpretations) and why he was excluded from the International Psychoanalytic Association. Knowing what your analyst will do will never be proof of anything, even when the patient takes it as proof of love.

Beyond these authors, Freud is perhaps the true inventor of the acephalic subject, the headless subject that orchestrates his disappearance. He elevates the subject not as the thinking subject, nor as the subject firm in their belief of having been loved, but as the subject who is eclipsed by the other and inhabited by a foreign body. In a moment I consider Lacan's eulogy to Freud, at the end of his paper on psychoanalytic technique, "The Direction of the Treatment and the Principles of Its Power" from 1958, one can find these death rings haunting us with the problem of interminable analysis.

"Who was more able than him," Lacan asks, "when avowing his dreams, to spin the thread on which the ring that unites us with being slides, and makes its brief shine glow in closed hands, passing it from one to the other in the swiftly shifting game of human passions?" (2006, 536). The ring isn't the ring of a secretly elected committee but, instead, the ring that ties our being to the thread of the unconscious upon which it slides, causing it to glow, swell, flash before our eyes. When it slides, we disappear.

The analyst isn't the one who knows nor the one who has the ring—nor the one who has the ring to give in the first place—but rather the one who knows how to close his hands upon this ring for a brief time in order to make it glow in the tumultuous game of human love and human passion. If the parodic church of the psychoanalytic initiates is an image of stasis and death, Lacan here gives us an image of psychoanalysis as pure movement. A game, perhaps a child's game, but serious as all children's games are. Lacan reads a movement into Freud's work that is the same movement implied by the drive and the process of analysis, a movement Lacan elevates against the Freudian movement, the institution of psychoanalysis.

"Who as fearlessly as this clinician, so firmly rooted in the everydayness of human suffering, has questioned life as to its meaning—not to say that it has none, which is a convenient way of washing one's hands of the matter, but to say that it has only one, that in which desire is borne by death?" (536). The meaning of suffering in the link between desire and death, especially insofar as it inheres in the splitting or *fault* of the subject—the last paper Freud wrote before he died—is eternal, infinite, and will not be overcome. The analyst can only add the word "nothing" to it. Nothing will change it. Lacan twists the "better not to have been born" of Oedipus toward the negative image of Freud's encounter with the three fates: born from nothing, good for nothing, returning again to nothing.

This is not pessimism or nihilism, nor is it some call for libertine indulgence or existential dread. It is merely a recognition of what there is, an acknowledgment of what exists. To put it paradoxically, in the spirit of Lacan's conclusion about women in his anxiety seminar: nothing is wanting from the position of the one who desires. What you cannot do, you can leave. The analyst is the one whose desire goes beyond the three fates, especially beyond their three concomitant fears: fear of the loss of the object, fear of the loss of the object's love, and fear of superego punishment. Each of these, in its own way, will, by the end of analysis, amount to nothing really—a signifier or series of signifiers, a memory or fantasy, family mythology and human suffering common to us all, as we grapple with what it means to have a body.

If the passions for Lacan are love, hate, and ignorance, it is the transformation of the analyst's relationship to knowledge—more than love and hate—that is decisive. This is a transformation that leaves the analyst in the position of the one who knows how to disappear *in* desire. Despite the stigmata left behind in the field of psychoanalysis by Freud and Lacan, I think it is the conversion of the analyst's relationship to knowledge and ignorance that accounts for what it means to be a psychoanalyst. If the analyst does not have some radical encounter with nonknowledge, this gift of nothing that embodies the link between desire and death, Lacan says quite categorically, he cannot be an analyst: "The positive fruit of the revelation of ignorance is non-knowledge, which is not a negation of knowledge, but rather its most elaborate form. The candidate's training cannot be completed without some action on the part of the master or masters who train him in this nonknowledge—failing which he will never be anything more than a robotic analyst" (297). It is the change that allows the analyst to disappear into a desire that can guide a treatment. This is at the heart of psychoanalysis: its conversion disorder.

The psychoanalyst's acts turn on this libidinal transformation—the only place where Lacan says the analyst will find anything worth saying at all to one's patients. If there is a fear, it is a fear of this transformative gesture: this sliding of the ring, the movement of nothing, the space of the body that will never be a knowledge, only an edge—all of which calls forth immense anxiety. The strange structuring of time in an unknown past and an unknowable future, which together ushers in the present, requires something from the analyst, even at minimum an act of surrender. At the other end, it brings with it the act of interpretation, the act of the analyst par excellence. Every interpretation leans on the analysis of the analyst, not in some narcissistic projection onto the patient but at the place where the signifier, this bodily event in the repetition of the transference, can be touched. Interpretation leans on the analyst's conversion.

Interpretation, then, is not some sort of active commentary or a conscious reconstruction of a veridical truth. It is something that takes root in the analyst's being—in a place where he does not know and does not think—condensing a moment of truth in being true to both patient and analyst. "An 'I do not think' which is the law, de facto," Lacan states, "makes the psychoanalyst depend on the anxiety of knowing where to give it its place in order to still think about psychoanalysis without being doomed to miss it" (1967–1968, 200). Here, we learn a little more about why Freud, as he rearranged his entire theoretical edifice, added to conversion disorder and its characteristic lack of anxiety an "I do not know" and an "I will not think about it," restoring repression's stature, making it the hallmark of an achievement, of having propelled oneself into the embodied passion of the symptom.

We also know why Freud repeated the foundational truth of faulty action at the end of his life, handing over his half-analysis to his daughter as an "I do not know what I am doing" that could have been taken up by her, by all of us, rather than playing into the desire for knowledge, especially the desire for the knowledge of the analyst. "But I never wanted to give anyone anything in the first place," Freud comically insists! Isn't that the fundamental truth of what it means to be an analyst, to be stuck in this impossible profession? Freud's desire is not only in question; it is put into question again and again, as an interminable *bis*! Encore!

XII

THE ANALYST'S ANALYSIS

Nothing's frugal. As for us, we want to give the city what lust has never ceased to put together. Young women or other women carrying their lovely voices as if on platters, their ten voices or nine voices in urgent errand dictating the imagination of matter.

It is not our purpose to obscure the song of no-knowledge.

—LISA ROBERTSON, *MAGENTA SOUL WHIP*

THE ANALYST'S ANALYSIS

If psychoanalysis hinges on the analysis and continued analysis of every analyst—what I am loosely calling the conversion of the psychoanalyst—what is to be done with its institution and training? What place does training hold in the conversion disorder of psychoanalysis? What needs to be transmitted, and how? I think that we must admit that, with regards to these questions, there is something rotten in the state of Denmark. Jacques Lacan is one of the only post-Freudian analysts to take up this question in any depth. His hope for the institution sprang from his return to Freud, and by reading Freud he found a sense of what in psychoanalytic experience must be transmitted not only in a training analysis but in the training of analysts.

This training experience cannot be separated from reading and writing, which is crucial to the transformation of every analyst. Freud founds the discipline of psychoanalysis by writing a dream book that takes flight from his self-analysis and his work with patients. In the best psychoanalytic writing, something happens so that some aspect of how the analyst works—with the drive, with sex, with the body—is transmitted beyond the mere knowledge put before the reader. Reading psychoanalysis can be a psychoanalytic and erotic experience. Thus, the transmission of psychoanalysis is wholly different from either the manual technique of surgeons, let's say, or the knowledge-cum-pedagogy of the philosopher. How?

Let me turn back to Lacan's article "Variations on the Standard Treatment," written in 1953. He asks a question about the modification of the ideal in the analyst's analysis and then turns to a question of training. This paper is written at a moment when Lacan's variations on the institutionalized version of Freudian treatment were under intense scrutiny, and, during this period, he was hiding his practice of varying session length. This paper attests to why he practiced the way he does, well before he was thrown out of the International Psychoanalytic Association. For me, this means that the paper lacks the pathos that followed his "excommunication," as he liked to call it.

Here he speaks powerfully about how the conversion of the analyst patient into the analyst proper happens, indicating the necessity for converting our relation to knowledge for the sake of analytic technique. This transformation requires that we wrest our ideals from the harsh grip of the superego.

Lacan claims that just because the ideal belongs to the imaginary "does not mean that it is illusory" (2006, 290). In fact, if one looks at imaginary numbers in mathematics or at an ideal point in geometry, it acts as "the pivotal point of transformation," a nodal point in a "convergence" of forms and figures determined *by* reality, not against it (290). This ideal is not inside any given thing or person but is a point of encounter with the outside that condenses subjective coordinates. Lacan speaks about finding the center of an ellipse, which has no center but is nevertheless structured by two foci from which an ideal point emerges, an imaginary or ideal center. This idea has been recognized by almost all tenets of psychoanalysis—from Klein to the ego psychologists and others—where something of the ideal as a structure of the ego must be transformed for an analysis to end. In this transformation, we can seek the future of psychoanalysis as a profession. Here, in relation to a question about the ideal, we can ask a crucial question about what an analyst knows and what must be transmitted from one analyst to another. How does an ideal work within our field?

Lacan states that although the analyst does not know what he is doing and changes "nothing in 'reality,'" psychoanalysis nevertheless "changes everything for the subject" (290). What does this mean about what the analyst changes? For one thing, it resists any idea of analytic conversion as a change in reality. Terms like "distortion of reality," "wishful thinking," and "magical thinking" as things to be corrected by analysis are not at the core of transformation for Lacan. They are simply, he says, an "excuse for ignorance" (290). Terms like "distortion" or "wishful thinking" often index the analyst's imaginary power to determine what is and isn't reality—his knowledge considered as a privileged point—exploiting the naïve faith of the patient who sees him as a man "not like the others" (290), a man who can give him the dose of reality that he was lacking. But what reality? Or rather, whose? Lacan is clear that this cannot be the ideal that the psychoanalytic institution transmits. It is a version of psychoanalysis sans conversion, mirroring the ideal of any moment in history, defining the real as rational and throwing the body under the sign of repression, doing away with the unconscious.

Once we ask who determines the outlines of a supposed reality, namely, the construction of a fantasy around a certain ideal, we get closer to the nodal ideal point of any imaginary form, closer to deconstructing this imaginary in the direction of something more material and, perhaps, Real in the Lacanian sense. Lacan's infamous example of this can be found in his reading of Freud's "A Child Is Being Beaten" in his 1966–1967 seminar *The Logic of Fantasy*. In the imaginary masturbatory scene of a father figure beating children, there is often a hidden instrument—a horse whip, a paddle with engravings, or an ivory cane—that is written with significance while it is invested with a material power. It is here where it is felt. The subject is indicated by this ideal point, saturated by symbolic content and material pleasure. At this critical place, the subject can reconstruct the unconscious fantasy—*I am being beaten by my father*—situating a state of excitement that had been warded off. Importantly, signification is intertwined with the excited and terrified body more than with a specified prior traumatic scene, which, in any case, is usually easily remembered in the case of masturbation fantasies. So while it is at the place of the ideal that we can find the subject and reconstruct the fantasy, it is also there where the body reveals itself.

Lacan breaks off this discussion of "reality" and returns to his claim that the analyst supports speech because it is there, at the place of the ideal, that speech must be supported—*I am being beaten by my father*. Suddenly Lacan asks the question: What is speech? He is immediately in the contradictory and somewhat tautological position of explaining what speech is with speech, saying the meaning of meaning. The discourse grows a little delirious—speech is not reducible to meaning, and meaning is not reducible to speech. However, speech does "give meaning its medium in the symbol that speech incarnates through its act . . . it is thus an act and, as such, presupposes a subject" (351). The word "incarnation" is important. Speech incarnates the subject it presupposes.

The speech act is on the side of the subject, and Lacan calls this "true speech," while "true discourse" is based in knowledge as "correspondence to the thing." In other words, speech that says "I" and speech that says "that." Speech that says "I" constitutes a truth the less it is based on true discourse and the more it is based on a subject's investment. True discourse is constituted as knowledge of reality outside the intersubjective dimension. The problematically egoic position of the analyst becomes an investment in true discourse at the expense of true speech. "That's the way it is," split off from its other half, "because that's the way I say it is." Lacan seems to think it would be better for analysts to announce their authority—"what I want to say to you is what I am saying; when I say stop, for example, you leave"—if that's what they need to do, and then let the patient reply, "I'm not leaving." This would be better than the ruse of pretending to interpret a patient's refusal to leave as something that doesn't implicate the analyst, displacing the intersubjective into some shadow from the past—"you don't want to leave because you want to stay and be beaten by me like your father once beat you." The patient should reply, "if I didn't want to leave, now I do."

Lacan calls this bifurcation of speech the "inter-accusation" of speech, and it acts like the Scylla and Charybdis the analyst must navigate. One always accuses the other of lying. Freud, in *Jokes and Their Relation to the Unconscious* ([1905b] 1995), in a section on skeptical jokes, acknowledges this division in speech with the famous joke of the two Jews who keep asking why the other one is lying about where he is going, to the point of delirium—"If you say you're going to Cracow, you want me to believe you're going to Lemberg. But I know that in fact you're going to Cracow. So why are you lying to me?" Freud goes on to say that these jokes form a special category of skeptical jokes.

> But the more serious substance of the joke is the problem of what determines the truth. The joke, once again, is pointing to a problem and is making use of the uncertainty of one of our commonest concepts. Is it the truth if we describe things as they are without troubling to consider how our hearer will understand what we say? Or is this only Jesuitical truth, and does not genuine truth consist in taking the hearer into

> account and giving him a faithful picture of our own knowledge? ...
> What they are attacking is not a person or an institution but the certainty of our knowledge itself, one of our speculative possessions.
>
> (115)

The joke about lying plays with an ineradicable uncertainty that comes from the division between Jesuitical and genuine truth. By playing on the uncertainty of truth in speech, the certainty of knowledge in general is under siege.

True discourse accuses true speech of lying because it points to the promise embedded in any declaration: pledging a future that belongs to no one. Ambiguity is always present because the future outruns the speaking person in question, who is always "outstripped." One can always accuse another person of lying. When someone says "I love you," the retort is often, as the famous song goes, "and what about tomorrow?" One has to say "I love you" again and again and again. On the side of true speech, questioning true discourse for what it signifies leads from one signification to another, then another. "What do you mean when you say you love me?" "What do you love about me?" "When did you decide you loved me?" And so on. Lover's discourse cannot catch up to the thing. "True discourse seems to be doomed to error" (Lacan 2006, 292). This is most apparent in the unending questions of children (why is the sky blue, what is air, who made air, what is time, how do you know, and so on), which lead back to an ur-question: why is the parent is answering the child's questions to begin with? In other words, we must ask a question about the position the parent occupies as the one who supposedly knows, returning us to this ideal point hidden inside knowledge.

This struggle in speech—working by way of ruses, trickery, error, and ambiguity—nonetheless stabilizes itself intersubjectively through conviction, agreement, or the stasis of continued battle. For Lacan, however, there is a difference between recognizing these structural laws, working with them, and the way in which we get lost in speech amid the struggle for power, especially in "the discourse of conviction, due to the narcissistic mirages that dominate" there (292).

It is a common trope that when a patient insists on how great we are or how they aren't angry with us in the slightest for cancelling their session, they mean precisely the opposite in their unconscious. "You are great" = "I hate you." The mirages of narcissism must be transparent to the analyst so that he or she does not take this utterance at face value and bask in a sense of greatness. However, an insistence on one's knowledge of the "I hate you" still participates in a mirage of narcissism. The analyst has to support the patient's coming to say "I hate you" for such and such particular reason.

How does this support of authentic speech happen? Lacan begins with a rather bleak pronouncement: authentic speech is forbidden to the patient except in rare moments of one's existence—hence the need for psychoanalysis. Nevertheless, it speaks and can be read in one's very being at "all the levels at which it [speech] has shaped him" (293). Lacan again grounds the work with the patient in an intersubjective foundation at the level of speech, a foundation that can be read by the psychoanalyst. The analyst must "silence the intermediate discourse in himself in order to open himself up to the chain of true speech, so that he can interpolate his revelatory interpretation" (293). To make sense of this cryptic but absolutely crucial statement, I will turn to Lacan's reading of Freud's case of the Rat Man.

Lacan argues that Freud solves the riddle of the Rat Man's obsessional neurosis in opening himself up to a "word chain" that unpacks the Rat Man's history, providing "the meaning by which we can understand the simulacrum of redemption that the subject foments to the point of delusion in the course of the great obsessive trance that leads him to ask for Freud's help" (293). The Rat Man came to Freud because he couldn't stop thinking of a torture method involving rats (described to him by his cruel captain in the army) that would be performed on his father and his lady love if he wasn't able to repay a small debt owed for his eyeglasses. Through a series of tricks driven by obsessional logic, he landed himself with the impossible duty of paying back Lieutenant A by paying back Lieutenant B. His father also happened to be dead, which somehow didn't prevent the possibility of rat torture in the afterlife.

Following the logic of this delusional "simulacra" of redemption, Freud traced the word "*Raten*"/rats to "*Ratten*"/installments, through a series of associations circling around an unpaid gambling debt of his father's from his days in the army, a debt that eventually led to his discharge. The Rat Man's unconscious accusation concerned a monetary/characterological problem of his father, who ended up marrying the Rat Man's mother for money and not the woman he loved. This cast a shadow over the whole of his parent's marriage, and at the point that the Rat Man fell ill, his mother was hypocritically asking the Rat Man to make a similar "calculation" when choosing a wife. In other words, she was asking him to marry a woman for wealth, not love. This forced the Rat Man into a fate similar to that of his parents—a kind of reverse Oedipus complex. Lacan points out that in his symptom, the Rat Man unites the real Oedipal couple, his father and his lady love, demonstrating his desire to marry the woman he loves and not obey his mother's injunctions to repeat his family history.

This chain unpacked by Freud is in fact not made up of "pure events (all of which had, in any case, occurred prior to the subject's birth), but rather of a failure (which was perhaps the most serious because it was the most subtle) to live up to the truth of speech and of an infamy more sullying to his honor" (293). This is incredibly important because questions of trauma and truth still haunt psychoanalysis. Truth, in this case, differs from veridical truth as "real" events; it is rather what Lacan would call subjective truth. Furthermore, the father and the lady love are precisely the nodal point of transformation in the case, a point where two narcissistic ideal images are subverted—the two besieged by the rats'/installments'—"undoing this chain in all its latent import," "summoning the subject," "less as a legatee than as its living witness" (294). The image is undone and reveals another body: one bored into, holding to an enjoyment even after death, an unmistakable desire for children, the Rat Man's passion for his father and lady love.

The Rat Man was forced to bear witness to a truth about his family, a truth that precedes his very birth, leaving its stamp on his body. In pointing out that the Rat Man is more witness than a legatee, Lacan indicates that analysis gives him back a choice regarding this legacy; in other words, the Rat Man is brought to a point where he can live up to his truth. This nodal point acts like a symbolic debt, something owned and assumed, though ultimately unfulfillable. The truth must be lived with and is opposed to its incarnation as a real debt, which can be simply paid off. Think here of his presenting problem of a delirious need to pay off the debt for his glasses. The Rat Man goes on to marry the woman he loves, sadly just before dying in the war.

Most important with regard to psychoanalytic technique and training is the fact that Freud was able to touch on this crucial point because a "similar suggestion" was made to Freud himself by his family and proved critical in his self-analysis. Lacan posits that if Freud had not rejected this decree by his own family and analyzed his relationship to money as it circulated in his family mythology, he may have missed it in the Rat Man. Presumably this is because he would have had to blind himself to his failed choice and its continued consequences, upholding the mirage dictated by his family.

While the effect of Freud's narcissism in his clinical work is a subject of much investigation—especially in the Dora case—still, Lacan says, "the dazzling comprehension Freud demonstrates . . . allows us to see that, in the lofty heights of his final doctrinal constructions, the paths of being were cleared for him" (294). Freud's self-analysis worked, and it is precisely this that allows Freud to slide down the signifying chain and read the Rat Man's story.

We now know that when Freud was writing his notes on the case, he wrote "Gisela Fluss!!!" with three unexplained exclamation marks. Either he means to indicate that this is a slip, a faulty action, because the Rat Man's Gisela cannot be Freud's Gisela Fluss—Freud's first passionate love, at the age of fifteen, who makes her appearance in Freud's 1899 "Screen Memories" paper and whose vibrant yellow dress forever affected him. Or, uncannily, they have the same exact name. In both cases, whether their lovers have the same name or it is in fact just a slip of the pen—my Gisela for your Gisela—the young lady in question for Freud is important.

Gisela is the woman from the country who he imagined would have provided him with a much richer life in his family-romance fantasy. She embodies, in a hallucinatory fashion, sexual satisfaction, deflowering, and having all the bread or money you need. This is Freud's family mythology hovering over an abyss: the myth that if they hadn't lost money and been forced to leave the country for the city, his life would have been splendid! All accounts would have been settled. Gisela names the undoing of some imagined injury or fall, a doppelganger for incestuous desire. The color yellow and this yearning for the satisfaction of country bread embody Freud's adolescent passion driven to a particular pitch, which was followed by depression, both of which were transformed into compulsive reading and the hoarding of books. These got him into trouble as a young man: Freud, much to his father's consternation, went into debt for buying too many books.

Lacan's point is deepened: It is not simply knowing the outlines of the fraught dynamics of family mythology pulling against a forbidden desire, nor is it the fantasy of escaping death in halfhearted attempts at sublimation; it is the singular crossing of Freud's analysis with his patient's, inherent in the slip or uncanny coincidence of this name Gisela. While this points to the importance of a close reading of Freud's cases, it also brings us back to the discussion of the analyst's knowledge— "namely, the contrast between the objects proposed to the analyst by his experience and the discipline necessary to his training" (294).

With regard to the question of analytic training, Lacan says that we know that malaise reigns. Lacan points us to Dr. Knight's 1952 address to the American Psychoanalytic Association, titled "The Present Status of Organized Psychoanalysis in the United States." While Knight characterizes the problems as those typical of a quickly growing institution, we know today that the same institution, without such numbers of new members, continues to have the same problems of malaise and infighting. In a section on professional standards and training, Knight characterizes the situation: "the spectacle of a national association of physicians and scientists feuding with each other over training standards and practices, calling each other orthodox and conservative or deviant and dissident, is not an attractive one, to say the least" (1953, 210).

Lacan quotes Knight at length concerning changes not only in training—from a program structured around a master figure to one resembling the structured bureaucracy of a medical school—but also in trainees, namely, from self-motivated introspective theoretical and well-read individuals to anti-intellectual, professionally hasty clinicians:

> It is quite clear, in this highly public discourse, how serious the problem is and also how poorly it is understood, if it is understood at all. What is desirable is not that the analysands be more "introspective" but rather that they understand what they are doing; and the remedy is not that institutes be less structured, but rather that analysts stop dispensing predigested knowledge in them, even if it summarizes the data of analytic experience.
>
> (Lacan 2006, 295)

This is one of the most direct criticisms and recommendations for training you will find in Lacan's oeuvre. The question of knowledge is central—even fundamental—when considering the experience of the analyst and his training. Analysts must stop dispensing predigested knowledge to patients and in their institutes. This has nothing to do with being "reflective," nor of cleansing reality of infantile wishes, nor even of being able to "go with the flow." Rather, it is about a transformation in one's ideals that brings about a transformation in the analyst's relation to knowledge.

Psychoanalytic training is not about the transmission of knowledge. Whether the experience of training happens via the candidate's experience in analysis, supervision, or an experience with teachers who know not to fetishize knowledge, it is about a revelatory encounter with ignorance essential to being a psychoanalyst. To take this one step further, I center this revelation on an experience of the body in transference as the conversion experience of psychoanalysis.

Most of the knowledge that analysis has accumulated, Lacan posits, is a "natural history of the forms of desire's capture and even of the subject's identifications," and these had never before been this rigorously catalogued (296). But this is not useful as a program for action on the part of the analyst. Because depicting the capture of desire in true discourse is notoriously difficult—as it is about the truth of illusion and the limits of illusion, which are never stable—it is also of little help to the analyst, since it concerns the deposit and not the mainspring. In other words, this knowledge does not concern what generates the world of the imaginary, what constructs the veil—that is, what creates the ideal.

The main bifurcation in post-Freudian theory concerning this mainspring has always been divided between biologizing drive theorists, on the one hand, and cultural humanists, on the other. Both suffer from problematic ideals seen in their respective idea of "drive harmony based on individualist ethics" and Darwin's science or humanist ideals of group conformity, which Lacan calls the covetousness of "engineers of the soul." Drive harmony holds little water when one takes into account the unhappy fault or splitting of the Freudian subject. In any case, the point of drives is disharmony. On the other hand, an orthopedic vision of the cultural sublimations of one's wounds also offers very little advantage. Psychoanalysis is best when subordinated to its unique purpose: its desire to convert a piece of reality by way of the symptom. The ideal is already this conversion in the frozen form of the bodily symptom.

Freud says that psychoanalysis is a science that puts itself into question with every new case. Every case should question what psychoanalysis thinks it knows. Imagine the modesty and flexibility of the analyst! This dictum clearly indicates for Lacan the path that training should follow: predigested knowledge will be of no help when analyzing a case. The analyst cannot analyze unless he "recognizes in his knowledge the symptom of his own ignorance" (296). He cannot be guided by any ideal. The ideal must be transformed into the material, given back its body, to allow the analyst to dispense with ideals and encounter the patient.

The desire to know is a symptom, maybe even *the* symptom, and it must be treated like the neurotic's desire to be loved, which is what the "best analytic writers" point to when they say the reason for becoming an analyst must be analyzed. Lacan refers the reader in a footnote to Maxwell Gitelson's 1954 article "Therapeutic Problems in the Analysis of the 'Normal' Candidate"—now a legendary paper—where he specifically takes up the challenge of Dr. Knight's address and the new ecology of candidates.

Gitelson says that the candidate's professionalism is the first line of an intellectual defense such that the imago of authority is now psychoanalysis itself, which makes it hard to analyze. Indeed, even when candidates sincerely affirm their intellectual acceptance of analysis, their normalcy works as a denial of the unconscious, especially their phallic ambition, which is an oral substitute and a defense against regression. They thus have great difficulty in "surrendering" to the uncertain gratification and postponed solutions demanded by analysis, and unfortunately the current analytic training system fosters these defensive solutions in its system of codified knowledge and struggle for power. This is especially true when the analysis of candidates, the so-called training analysis, is seen as a learning process distinct from therapy or regular analysis, in other words, as dealing in a transmission of knowledge between a teacher and a student.

We come back to the "closing" of the unconscious predicted by Freud in the 1920s as the turning point of analytic technique, linked to the potential effects of analysis becoming more widespread. "Indeed the unconscious shuts down insofar as the analyst no longer 'supports speech,' because he already knows or thinks he knows what speech has to say" (Lacan 2006, 297). The patient cannot recognize his truth in what the analyst says, because there is no revelation, or new encounter, nothing that strikes the surface of his body. This is the surprising effect not only of what Freud says to a patient but also its status as a truth for Freud—one he encountered in his own analysis.

True speech must be true for both parties, united *in* the interpretation. This is a quite radical point and one not often addressed in the literature on technique. It puts at the center the necessity of the analyst's analysis as an experience of the unconscious as well as the rediscovery of the coordinates of a truth in the coming-to-say of interpretation. Speech reveals an unconscious subject, and it can only do so by following the vicissitudes of the body in the act of saying.

Interpretation must be as surprising to the analyst as it is to the patient, as if what the analyst said literally fell out of his or her mouth, as if the analyst's body procured this speech quite without the analyst. Lacan's emphasis on oracular speech resonates here, with the added element of a lack of knowledge or intention. The analyst rediscovers his or her specificity in a new form in every case, with every interpretation. This avowal by the analyst, the use of the analyst's body, which acts even in silence, allows patients to find themselves *in* the analyst. While this might risk being nothing more than a narcissistic identification on the part of the analyst, remaining on the threshold of bodily tension in the act of saying prevents this. Work with the materiality of saying is the antidote to identification and narcissism.

Lacan points out that narcissism is always the rejection of the commandments of speech as linked to the body and that one would see in an analysis caught in the analyst's narcissism the ferocious reign of the superego, opened up to the solidification of the imaginary away from the life of the drives. The body does not tolerate this well. I have often been a patient's second (or third or fourth) therapist, and while some symptoms might have resolved, their superegos are as harsh as ever, especially in their discourse about themselves as symptomatic—"I have such and such problem, and it is for this and this reason." They are almost thoroughly objectified, their bodies revolting from a diagnosis they will never recognize, usually by dispensing with pleasure first.

No judgment—usually partaking of the good/bad variety—can stabilize the subject. This instability, this vanishing point, is preferable to the avid stability of an objectified self. The subversion of the superego in the direction of its vanishing is also necessary on an institutional level, Lacan claims, if psychoanalysis is going to function. In this paper from 1953, "Variations on the Standard Treatment," that vanishing must take place on the plane of knowledge. Here we are given the bidirectional coordinates of treatment: speech and the body on the one hand, the imaginary and the superego on the other.

Lacan then enters into one last parody of the modern-day analyst. Here the analysand in training analysis confirms his knowledge of his Oedipal problems by confessing that he is in love with the woman who opens the door to his sessions, who he believes is his analyst's wife. Lacan quips that this titillating fantasy is just conformism and is hardly a lived knowledge of Oedipus, which would strip him entirely of this fancy because it is nothing but the road of total undoing. This is not how Oedipal desire appears in an analysis; there it is a bodily eruption surrounded by a field of anxiety.

"A hundred mediocre psychoanalysts do not advance analytic knowledge one iota" (296), Lacan declares. There is nothing but the desire for analysis, for the psychoanalysis to carry on, for the psychoanalysis to be psychoanalysis and not something else. The analyst must find a position that allows her to sustain this desire. Only if we understand this, he says, will we understand Freud's discretion when he says: "I must however make it clear that what I am asserting is that this technique is the only one suited to my individuality; I do not venture to deny that a physician quite differently constituted might find himself driven to adopt a different attitude to his patients and to the task before him" (300). Lacan points out that this is not a sign of Freud's profound modesty—some sort of idealization of Freud that masks profound aggression—but instead points to a truth about the analyst's relation to knowledge.

The analyst must know that she cannot proceed by mimicking Freud, which would only be formalistic. Instead, she should find her scale of measurement along the path of nonknowledge. To take this one step further, Lacan implies that every analyst must reinvent psychoanalysis, must invent his or her own being, attitude, and way as an analyst. Freud leaves this open—demands it, even. Is this not the conversion of the analyst? Turning neurosis into a way of working and listening? The standard treatment decrees variation, this individual variation as an invention of oneself as an analyst, because you can only be your own being, your own body—which if you haven't found a way with by the time you make your way into the analyst's chair, you will be lost, and you will always be lost. There is no other way to navigate with the unconscious.

To end, let me tell you about another dream, close in form to Lacan's analysis of Freud and the Rat Man. It is a late dream, a product of self-analysis, that delimits the incestuous familial field; in some sense it's too revealing, in another, too banal to reveal much of anything, but still, it shows something critical about the work of an analyst's analysis. The dream began with the phrase—*the psychoanalytic institution has forgotten the world, and the world has forgotten the psychoanalytic institution*—which was conveyed to me by the attempt to build a transatlantic tunnel that couldn't complete itself. Recently, I had been in the subway with my son in Washington, DC, there for the Women's March, and we had marveled at their train stations' round structure. I spoke with him about how subways all look different in different cities—a fact easily forgotten by egocentric New Yorkers. We talked about how fun it must be for a city to decide on the architectural aesthetics of their subway.

After catching a glimpse of this half-completed tunnel, the scene changed to a thrift store, where a friend was showing me old miniature paintings by masters, which seemed to cost and be worth hundreds of thousands of dollars. I had the desire to steal one but resisted. After having taken the back off of one to examine the construction of the painting, perhaps to assess whether it was real, the painting got lost in the shuffle. I was only left with the frame. I was terrified that I wouldn't be able to prove my innocence if caught, since I had in fact wanted to steal it, but then I began to doubt myself. Had I in fact stolen it?

The scene changes again, and I am with my stepmother. It is revealed that she has been stealing money from my father, that they live quite separately, and that he was in fact quite alone, as she lives in the Caribbean now. Suddenly, I am being told that my father has died and that I must go to the hospital to make arrangements, but the term used is "grampy," or what my son calls my father, and it is my father telling me. It is as if he has split into two people, father/grampy. I am told that I have inherited an office that I can use for my psychoanalytic practice, but when I go to visit this office (and not my dead father), my second analyst (who bears my father's mother's name) is the person who runs the building. I wonder if this is an appropriate arrangement, and the dream ends.

When I woke up, I realized that the "proper" Oedipal parental couple had been created by the dream—Grampy and my analyst—a couple I never knew, since my father's father had died tragically when my father was a child. In fact, my mother's father also died tragically when my mother was a child—probably the real reason they married each other, this problem with the loss of fathers—so I never had a grandfather. My mother's mother never remarried and raised eight children alone. My father's mother remarried, but this husband also died suddenly not long after they were married and then never remarried. My parents, after they divorced, married younger spouses that never had children, and so one could say that there was never an intact family: a fact of my particular heritage but also something linked to the Depression, immigration, and war.

In creating the lost parents of my parents through my analyst, the dream points to the destruction of the family, from which my parents never recovered and from which I, in ways, also have not. It points to the line of transgression: reminiscent of Freud's father in his experience at the Acropolis, who says to him, "be where I am and go no further." This point fuels the wish, the prohibition, and its place in a family-romance fantasy. This dream comes at a moment when I want to cross the line, steal what isn't supposed to belong to me, and was having great difficulty without knowing why.

It's funny that the dream is set off by this strange pronouncement about the psychoanalytic institution. God knows I am no fan of it, and I quickly saw through the family romance of the institution itself, even when I was seduced by it. The recognition of its shattered state seemed necessary for psychoanalysis to figure out how to be relevant again in a world that hadn't just turned against it, as they often like to imagine, but had completely forgotten it—something that seemed impossible to know as long as they held close to the romance with which they unethically seduced candidates.

I am some generational anomaly, the American Lacanian, the product of this incomplete transatlantic tunnel. It is true that I never go to Paris—as one analyst said to me once somewhat condescendingly: "when you told me you were a Lacanian from Miami, Florida, I thought, well, it's a whole new world." In a way, I knew and acted on all this first and left the institutional fold before I knew the entrenched place of "all of it" in my own life, in relation to my family history. Knew is an overstatement, I knew some; I know some now. This dream, on the other hand, crystallized something, perhaps not because of this alliance between my history and my formation as an analyst but because of working as an analyst. This is the frame that I have to work with.

The dream came on the heels of intense work with a patient whose child had died very late in a pregnancy. The mourning, as I'm sure you can imagine, was intense, probably the most intense I had been through with anybody. I caught a reaction in myself, something that I recognized as a reaction I have to severe trauma, in which I secretly blamed the person for what tragically befell them. I noted it and put it aside, but it returned in veiled form in what I came to say to her. I said that it was a terrible kind of fate, something that on the surface might seem dangerous to say to a mother who has just lost a child—almost saying to her that it was bound to happen. The reason I could say it, or did, was because her mother had abandoned a child in a family she had and didn't want, decimating that family before constituting the family she had with my patient, which remained intact. My patient could say very little about what this meant to her, though her life seemed to be guided by its figure, returning to the place where this other family lived again and again, ending up in tragic scenarios there.

She had seemingly taken a step out of this cycle of repetition when she lost the child, when she was there, again. The blame from me was directed at this uncanny repetition, this repetition that I thought the analysis should have stayed, as if I should have prevented this child from dying and didn't—so it must be her fault. Why did you go there! I wanted to scream at her. You know what we have talked about all these years! My patient, being less omnipotent than I imagined myself to be (and thus more psychoanalytic), said to me, "you are the only person who knows this and whom I can speak to about this. Maybe, having had to bury her there, I have made up for my mother's sins, I have given a child back, a child that left me and not I her, and I can finally leave all this behind." She put me back in my place as her psychoanalyst and took from the interpretation what was real beyond the pathos of my guilt and blame.

If all of this wasn't uncanny enough, my mother also lost a child late in a pregnancy, something that marked my birth, her abandonment of me, and the disintegration of my parent's marriage. In fact, I decided long ago that my first name bears this child in it—the son of James. More than this, her blame—whichever direction it went, to my father, to me— was already a displaced reaction and repetition in relation to the loss of her own father. My father's helplessness in the face of her, and of me, is part of his own repetition—left to take care of his mother, whose husbands kept dying. An unconscious economy of blame circulates as the melancholic family bond. This is how families are destroyed. All of this is as it is. The story in some sense is common, as common as a miscarriage, a divorce, a death, even if it sounds like the fated stories psychoanalysts like to tell. I don't think I like telling it.

All in all, the details are neither here nor there, except for the fact that I have to know this in myself to hear the patient—not to console, cover over, or blame but rather to find the words that allow her the space to say what she needs to say about having lost this child. The strange thing is that her transference to me always turned on a question of what she could allow herself to believe and whether I wanted her to believe what everyone else seemed to believe, which she could see but didn't believe, because it always seemed to be self-protective. And if I didn't want this, was I willing to leave her in a place where she believed nothing, or something painfully idiosyncratic? Certainly, this is how she has constructed the question about the desire of her mother and this other family. She also came to me for symptoms related to anxiety, especially concerning her body, which she saw as damaged and infertile, which evolved into this particular transference. It is true that the pregnancy was part of the analysis, of where it had brought her.

Through this tragedy, something in this deadlock of an either/or shifted. To my depiction of her tragic fate, she added the belief that she knew exactly when the baby died and her desire to tell people about this when they offered her the palliative care generally offered to grieving mothers. She could tell me, even if she can't tell others, because they don't want to hear it, and only I knew what it meant in the context of her history—everything she had been through in order to arrive here. There is an element of belief in all of this, insofar as both the moment of the baby's death and its place in her family history are constructed retrospectively—a private truth or belief that is nonetheless shared, refusing in psychoanalysis to screen out the worst. We can see the sexual bonds and the force of unbinding in families, against the affectionate delusion or myth of the family-romance fantasy. We do not have to proceed, even if we pay attention to politeness, pretending that everything is fine. It is not.

One of the last things she told me was that her phobic anxieties about this or that thing had strangely resolved. She had watched, without blinking, a video of an animal she found quite terrifying. Her other presenting symptom was that she couldn't feel things in her body, that there was this enigma concerning all that was inside of her, and a terror of what it looked like when it came out. With everything that she had to look squarely in the eye, this body forced into the outside, the nonfeeling of her body also fell away. After a period of time, after grieving, she told me she was looking forward to getting her body back—a somewhat inaccurate way of putting it, since it will have changed so much by the time it returns to her. This also meant the necessity of refinding a sense of sexuality again, one not simply tied to the life-and-death vicissitudes of procreation. But isn't this what she always had come to do? And wasn't the difficulty simply that it was tied in this way and needed to find a way to untie itself?

Psychoanalytic conversion appears like this: feverish, burning, splintering, stillborn, sick, paralyzed, bruised, shaking, and excited. My Gisela for your Gisela, my stupid name for your terrible tragedy, my pregnancy for yours, my body for your body. Who has the courage? Courage, after all, is not something found once and for all, nor is it not found, leaving one in the despair of anxiety or boredom. It is separate from us—there when it is allowed finally to be there where it wasn't a moment before. It is the name for an aptitude that psychoanalysis cultivates, which can appear when it needs to—like dreams, slips of the tongue, humor, and self-analysis. This conversion that brings you, as an analyst, to the place where you can use your body to separate from your patients at the place where it is most painfully joined.

Is psychoanalysis about the unfounded, about what is impossible to get your hands around and keep, aside from knowing something about the fact one's fate is sealed? Is this unfounded, half-formed, and half-said, the transformation of the sick body into an analytic body? The psychoanalytic institution, which wasn't founded by Freud, must find a way to mirror this destiny that becomes the fate of every analyst—to hold us together there. *The psychoanalytic institution has forgotten the world, and the world has forgotten the psychoanalytic institution.* I've come to know that I was never going to be anything else than a psychoanalyst, and, by virtue of this, I must learn to live with (what can only be called) my conversion disorder.

ACKNOWLEDGMENTS

An earlier version of the chapter "I Am Not a Muse" was published in *Division/Review* 15 (2016), reprinted with permission. Part of the chapter "Forged in Stones" was published as "Begin Again: On Forgetting, Repetition, and Atonement," *European Journal for Psychoanalysis* 3 (2015), as well as in *Lacan, Psychoanalysis, and Comedy* (2017), edited by Patricia Gherovici and Manya Steinkoler for Cambridge University Press, reprinted with permission. The chapter "How to Burn" is based on an op-ed I wrote in the *New York Times*, "The Accidents of Psychoanalysis," December 6, 2014.

I would like to acknowledge my faithful interlocutors, co-teachers, and simply beloveds, Todd Altschuler, Chiara Bottici, Marcus Coelen, Patricia Gherovici, Elissa Marder, Evan Malater, and David Lichtenstein—thank you for reading and rereading my work, which has always tried to live up to your own. I would also like to thank my editor, Wendy Lochner, who believed in this project, no less in the importance of psychoanalytic writing, and allowed me to do what I wished, a courage more and more rare, to which I must add my thanks for their unwavering support of this disordered book—Judith Butler, Jean-Michel Rabaté, and Mari Ruti. To my dear colleagues, thank you for making psychoanalytic work and theory an adventure when I need it most, which is often: Sergio Benvenuto, Felix Bernstein, Eliana Calligaris, Fernando Castrillon, Monique David-Ménard, Luce Delire, Susan Finkelstein,

Michael Garfinkle, Adrienne Harris, Ben Kafka, Kyoo Lee, Kelly Merklin, Kerry Moore, Michael Moskowitz, Carol Owens, Jason Royal, Eyal Rozmarin, Vladimir Saftle, Beatriz Santos, Cassandra Seltman, Marc Strauss, Vanessa Sinclair, Ceclia Wu. As well, my sincere thanks to my student editors, Anna Banker and Christina Lowe, who went above and beyond the call of duty. Some friends, some of whom are writers and others otherwise, or probably better, disposed in life, much love to you for your patience with my psychoanalytic banging on: Oliver Clegg, Shirley Cook, Alison Gingeras, Frank Haines, Javier Hernandez, Courtney Love, Jesse Pearson, Lybov Persev, Vanessa Place, Ashley Quaine, Alan Reid, Richard Smith, Rachel Valinsky, Sam West. Finally, my gratitude to my patients for teaching me every day about the courage to live with a body in this world.

APPENDIX

One week after turning in a draft of this book for final review to Columbia University Press, I was rushed into surgery for acute appendicitis. It is true that I had been messing around with my body: I was on an extended cleanse for over a month and was visiting various "healers," who were recommending nutritional and herbal supplements. All this, after one such person recommended the megaprobiotic that seems to have caused the peritonitis, exacerbated a weakness in an already belabored system. This was very much my own doing, even if I conscripted others into the performance.

I can't really say why I was doing it. The overriding concern seemed to be vanity, if I was going to try to be honest with myself, yet there was some uncontrollable curiosity about this world, which seeks to heal the body and is full of explanations for just about everything. I was playing at believing in it all—believing that gluten was evil and inflammation a contemporary malaise; that in the search for an elusive pH balance, my gut biomes were in need of major intervention; that only infrared saunas could take on this plague of toxins—I could go on and on. I wanted to believe, *and* I wanted to figure out what was ideological, as if the two could somehow be separated if I really gave myself over to the project and watched how I came out the other side.

The problem was that I began enjoying the ritualistic pleasure of it all, including the concreteness of the concerns. Yes! Any day now, I will become a new person. Every day, I could measure any number of factors and interpret waves of energy or excitement or lethargy as part of this massive process of transformation and these various self-administered cures. During the initial pains from the peritonitis, I insisted that I was merely in a "healing crisis"—that the pain was a sign of how toxic I was, reasserting the usefulness of my efforts. You begin to see the circular logic. You also begin to see what is crazy about this management and ministration of the body, whose only point, in some sense, is to test it, or break it, or both. All of this rationalization, until the moment that I felt the pain localize into that infamous area on the lower right known as McBurney's point (coined in 1889) and promptly went to the hospital.

Was this a way of dealing with this book, which needed finishing—for all that is horrifying about bringing a project to an end? A necessity for separation that took the form of a literal cut? Was it an addendum to my research about conversion disorder and the body? A hysterical sympathy for so many in a nearly insane quest for bodily purification? Did I need to lose an organ, even this supposedly useless or vestigial one? Maybe that is always the organ to lose? Or, if I was going to push the question at hand, perhaps we should admit that there is something dangerous about writing books because there is no metaposition—I am entirely inside the project of writing about somatic transformations and conversion disorder. The appendix was always going to cost me an appendix.

Perhaps you know, after reading this book, that the next question at this point is: what does any of this have to do with the sexual? Well, a lot. I was alone during this period of the summer, and this cleanse was how I spent my time as I raced to finish this book. Furthermore, some questions about getting older, my child becoming an adolescent, questions about children and family, were certainly on my mind. But, as with Freud, it is at this point in the analysis when discretion dictates that I go no further. What I can say is, after this whole fiasco, sitting in my hospital room recovering, I was reminded that Dora also had appendicitis—or rather, that a question of appendicitis had played a role in the ending of her treatment with Freud. This appendicitis was also a hysterical pregnancy.

The rediscovery of the appendicitis in the final sessions becomes the linchpin in Freud's sense of the point in an analysis where a hysterical symptom reveals its contact with an organic base. This place is where the sexual, as such, asserts itself, literally more than phantasmatically. We might remember that Freud's Dora case, titled "Fragment of an Analysis of a Case of Hysteria," was written as a supplement—or appendix—to *The Interpretation of Dreams*. This is why the work is not a traditional case presentation and is written as an elucidation of analysis as structured by two important dreams—hence the qualification of it as fragmentary. More than showing the place of dreams in a psychoanalytic cure, what we learn about (and what everyone remembers) is Freud's countertransference to Dora. The fragmentary is not only about the nature of dream work but the abrupt termination of the treatment by Dora. Not a whole case, a cut appendix.

It is in Dora's second and final dream, the dream that leads Dora to announce that she is leaving the treatment, that the appendicitis comes into the foreground. In this dream Dora finds a letter from her mother telling her that her father has died and that she can come home if she likes. After some train trouble, a situation that becomes a strange kind of sexual geography, mapping the feminine body through the topography of the train, the station, the woods, Dora arrives home to find everyone gone (probably to the cemetery) and settles down to read the big book on her writing table. It is in her associations to this big book that we find the link to appendicitis.

Dora recalls that at the time of her favorite aunt's illness, she received a letter that her cousin, her aunt's son, had fallen ill with appendicitis and that she should not come to visit. She had gone to look up the symptoms of appendicitis in a big book—an encyclopedia. Freud then recalled that after her aunt died some time later, Dora had an attack of appendicitis and recognized the special localization of pain that she had read about. Freud says this is the one symptom that he did not regard as a hysterical production because of the nature of the fever and the localization of the pain. Yet it seems worth noting that in the description of the appendicitis by Freud, there is a confusion between this acute illness in her bowels, her regular problems with constipation, and Dora's menstrual period, which arrived two days into her appendicitis attack and was itself accompanied by severe abdominal pains, all of which resolved. Strange.

Then, just as Freud is in the midst of describing the nature of the illness, reconsidering whether it was hysterical, he says he was about to abandon this entire track when Dora suddenly provided the key, "producing her last *addendum* to the dream" (263, italics mine): *"she saw herself particularly distinctly going up the stairs."* Just as Freud loses hope at the point of conversion, Dora will respond to him with an addendum. She tells Freud that after her attack of appendicitis, she had trouble walking—especially on stairs—and to this day still drags her foot. To which Freud cried, "Aha, the true hysterical symptom!" Neurosis, he says, seized upon a chance event to make use of it for its own purposes.

Dora's repartee to Freud's excitement is that the attack of appendicitis took place nine months after the famed sexual proposition by Herr K at the lake—her father's lover's husband—that brought her to analysis. So the hysterical pregnancy—a wished-for child—responded to the hystericizing events that brought Dora's world crashing down. It was at this moment that she left a letter for her parents to find that said she was going to commit suicide; they then brought her in to see the good doctor Freud.

Of course Freud goes on to use this hysterical pregnancy as further proof of Dora's love for Herr K, not only treating the symptom too metaphorically but adding to it his heterosexual bias. We now know that the story is a bit more complicated. The appendicitis-cum-pregnancy fantasy points back to the painting of the Sistine Madonna Dora had sat in front of, rapt, unable to move for two hours. This rapture is folded into this final dream, its sexual geography and her attempt to map the female body. For those who know the painting, it is one of the most sumptuous images of the baby Christ.

This quest is bound to Dora's attachment not to Herr K but to his wife, Frau K, her father's mistress. It was this same mistress with whom she had read about sexual matters in big books, a fact she hid from Freud for quite some time in the analysis, leaving him to wonder where she had gotten all of her sexual knowledge. Frau K, importantly, would go on to betray Dora mercilessly, giving to her husband his trump card when defending himself against Dora's accusations—saying that a girl who read such things in books would not have earned the interest of a man like him. Brutal.

Shouldn't we instead see Dora as attempting to restore her precious feminine desire through her hysterical pregnancy cum appendicitis—this point of desire that had been excoriated in a plot that involved everyone she loved? Is this not the desire that Frau K helped her keep moving by talking to her about men, her husband, Dora's father, sexual matters, and children, leading to their extraordinary intimacy, to say nothing of Dora's complicity with the strange familial arrangement where she distracted Herr K when Frau K was off with her father? Or perhaps better, isn't this one way of understanding hysterical pregnancy itself, the symptom situated at this point of collapse, when she cannot sustain an ideal any longer and must find support in the body? A place to prop herself up? Isn't the appendicitis like the nodal point of a web of complex identifications in the search for satisfaction with another? A point on the body that is literally her search for knowledge of femininity, for knowledge of bodies?

Even if this is the spider's web in which she is caught, it is a web she has woven, and the desire depicted in the final dream seems to be one of a separation—from her family. This is the place she had reached in her analysis through this persistent question about what a woman is and can have. Something of this feels palpably contained in her repeated use of the word "calm" in the dream. She sat down, by herself, calmly to read her big book. Yes, calm (*ruhig*) also means its opposite, excited—thank you, Freud—but it also means rest, as in final resting place, peace. Dora weaves together sexual excitement, death, mourning, and peace or rest to find herself separate from all these others, who are all overexcited, all enmeshed in one another's *jouissance*.

This is also something that Dora may also have found in Raphael's extraordinary depiction of the Madonna, whose face indicates her coming intimacy with loss. Freud, it must be said, stays very far away from this constellation. We know that he fails to take into account both the place of Dora's mother in the case, along with her homosexual desire for

Frau K. He also never inquires further about what captivated her in the painting of the Madonna, nor does he ask about her desire for a child. In the end, he takes what she has to say about dreaming of her father's death, being free of her parent's constraints, and the appendicitis attack as Dora wrestling not with separation but with a morbid craving for revenge.

His thoughts about her desire for revenge, her sadistic wishes, eclipse any consideration of Dora's attempt to acquaint herself with a more intimate knowledge of desire and death, desire and loss, especially as it wraps itself around her ill father, who is petrified of dying. Isn't this best seen in that amazing scene in association to her asking a hundred times—where is the train station?—when, in reality, she asks her mother five times—where is the key?—in order to fetch her father's brandy, recalling suddenly that when her father was given a toast that he may enjoy the best health for many years to come, she saw a strange quiver pass across his face? This is what she's calmly trying to read about in her big book.

Freud equates what Dora is reading about—"pregnancy, childbirth, virginity, and so on" (267)—with a pun on her own name found in another addendum to the dream, when she asks about her father, "Does Herr_ live here? Where does Herr_ live?" We now know that Dora's name is Ida Bauer, and *Bauer* is indeed an "ambiguous and improper word" with a whole series of meanings that move metonymically from farmer, to cage, to cave, to a room for women, habitat or home more generally, to enjoyment, masturbation, and finally semen. Indeed, where is the station? Where is the key? Does Herr Bauer live here? Incredible that the question is already present in Dora's name!

It is important for me that you know that I write all of this without wanting to belabor Freud's mistakes, as so many have. Freud had the uncanny ability to give us this incredible case, despite all of his faults. And, most importantly, I'm fascinated by the fact that the one symptom Freud "overlooked" turned out to be *the* hysterical symptom that was the linchpin in the conclusion of her treatment, that Freud throws his hands up in the face of this bodily element of conversion, just as he would twenty-six years later in *Inhibitions, Symptoms, and Anxiety*.

At the "real" somatic eruption (not her hysterical cough) that the neurosis seizes upon, we find the most condensed point of fantasy and the crystallization of Dora's response to her psychoanalysis, pushing Freud into what he can't understand about conversion, no less, working with female patients. Isn't there something powerful in the play by play of Dora and Freud around this appendicitis, everything that Freud couldn't understand at that time, allowing Dora finally to add some piece of her own knowhow? Don't we see clearly Dora's capacity to work in her counterassertions to Freud's bumbling analysis of her appendicitis? Think of her final remark, aimed at Freud's satisfaction in his concluding statements on her pregnancy fantasy and supposed love for Herr K—"Why, has anything so very remarkable come out?" Can't Freud just calm down a little?

I'd like to oppose this "nothing remarkable has come out" to the increasingly intensified localization seen at the place of her final conversion symptom, the sensation of peritonitis, but also by virtue of the images in the dream, Raphael's Sistine Madonna—her anguished face and that beautiful massive baby—and finally Dora's question that concerns her very name: where does Bauer live? As Freud noted, his analysis was going to take too long, especially if he carried on in the way he was, searching for the appendix to *The Interpretation of Dreams* through her. Dora has her sight fixed somewhere else—this cartography of the body, the attempt to localize something in response to her repeated question—where? Lacan has repeatedly said that even if Freud wasn't happy with her terminating him, she did leave the treatment in order to confront Herr K, Frau K, and her father with the truth, which restored some of her sense of dignity.

What, then, was I was returning to, in returning to this case—my appendicitis for Dora? My feeling is that it was something powerful about the mythical localization of pain in appendicitis that is also close to the localization of desire both in psychoanalysis and in the experience of pregnancy. This is where it hurts. This is what has transformed. Conversion does just this—localization is the work of the symptom, its feat of condensation, and the power of materialization. It is the perfect expression of desire—brought to the point of a precise problem, namely, feminine desire in all its bodily exigency. What else is pregnancy? This most glorified of all problems, the most visible indication of a woman's sexuality? Or, as they used to say about pregnant girls—she's in trouble.

Perhaps to conclude, we should note that the word "appendix" indicates the small outgrowth of an internal organ as well as the supplemental material at the end of a book. Both organ and writing. Coming from the Latin *appendere*, which means "to cause to hang," to suspend, it carries in it the meaning of appending, adding, subjoining, upending, as well as to weigh, pointing to the old method of weighing, as in hanging something by a string or thread. You can see this meaning in words that carry "pen" as in to draw out, carry, or spin: compendium, compensate, depend, pendulum, propensity, and so on.

Appendix indicates a relationship between two objects and the distance between two objects, as in span, or suspend; also to spin, as in to weave two threads together—to spin a web, to join, plait, or fasten together. In any case, doesn't all this point to my name—Webster—meaning weaver or spinster, a word that also serves as a derogatory term for a single or an old woman, possibly childless. Importantly, Webster as weaver, through appendix, traces the fact of separation that is behind every act of joining or appending, the very essence of a supplement. So even if this is a book on the body, we are never very far from the signifier. We simply can't forget how literally a signifier must be taken, including the way it moors itself in the body in order to respond to the hysterical question—where?—by marking, naming, externalizing, writing, and materializing. The ability to localize is the power of conversion symptoms—this special aptitude that writes itself into its own appendix.

NOTES

INTRODUCTION

1. The concept of the outside (*le dehors*) will be developed in subsequent chapters, in particular as an investigation into the psychoanalytic conception of the object, reading thinkers like Bachelard, Blanchot, Foucault, and Nancy with and against Lacan's concept of ex-sistence or extimacy (exterior intimacy). Lacan was critical of concepts of subjectivity as linked to interiority and used various topological models to show the subject as positioned on a kind of edge, with the object situated just beyond this threshold. His neologism—*extimacy*— uses Freud's concept of the uncanny to remind us that what is closest to home is always the most foreign and, more generally, that the unconscious acts like a foreign body or parasite on identity, seen most clearly in conversion hysterics.
2. Important in Freud's *Group Psychology and the Analysis of the Ego* (1921) is the dialectical relationship between neurosis and exile from group psychology. He calls any philosophical or religious mythology a "crooked" cure.
3. There are several thinkers of great importance to me concerning a conception of the post-Freudian era as ushering in a new sociological conception of the subject deemed therapeutic. See Rieff (1966).
4. See James ([1902] 1982).
5. This tautology of the conversion of conversion becomes important in reading the history of Freud and his use of the concept.

I. DAYBREAK

1. In Sandor Ferenczi's famous 1949 paper "The Confusion of Tongues Between the Adults and the Child (The Language of Tenderness and of Passion)," he speaks to the mismatched languages of adults and children, especially when it comes to sexuality.

Here the question isn't so much a question of abuse or trauma as a special instance but of the traumatic encounter more generally between these colliding worlds of tenderness and passion, childhood and adult sexuality and aggression.

2. In Lacan's 1967–1968 unpublished seminar *The Psychoanalytic Act*, the question of how psychoanalysis conceives of an act is of utmost importance, since presumably we help our patients act or at the very least see their failed acts, for example, slips of the tongue and bungled actions or mistakes, which Freud marked early on. Right away, Lacan contrasts the act we commit that we don't know about and what it means to be equal to one's action. He says that far from this being some autonomous rational decision making, psychoanalysis shows another possibility, a radical conversion in our relationship to knowing, acting, deciding. In this quotation, Lacan is asking a question concerning the danger of some psychoanalysts only going halfway in this "conversion," which he centers on a conversion in our relationship to the fantasy of absolute knowledge as what will make action possible.

3. In general, Lacan was interested in the comingling of symptoms, and certainly this goes back to his first psychiatric writings on the famous case of the Papin sisters and their psychotic *folie a deux*, which led them to murder their employer. But it is interesting to note that all love relationships, including that between analyst and patient, also take part in this symptom partnering.

4. Agamben's 1993 *The Coming Community* should be situated with a series of theoretical texts addressing the question of groups and community following Freud's *Group Psychology and the Analysis of the Ego* ([1921] 1995) as well as fascism and World War II more generally. Important are Blanchot's *The Unavowable Community* (1988) and Nancy's *The Inoperative Community* (1991). The idea of the irreparable and what is without remedy is important to Agamben in being able to see what exists outside the lens of either redemption or salvation, things as they are, and therefore situated historically. Only then can we understand what to change and what project might bind us together.

5. Freud can be found on a number of occasions lamenting the problems of woman's superego, which was somehow both too intact and too fragmented. Take, for instance, the following remarks from his paper "Some Psychical Consequences of the Anatomical Distinction Between the Sexes": "I cannot evade the notion (though I hesitate to give it expression) that for women the level of what is ethically normal is different from what it is in men. Their super-ego is never so inexorable, so impersonal, so independent of its emotional origins as we require it to be in men. Character-traits which critics of every epoch have brought up against women—that they show less sense of justice than men, that they are less ready to submit to the great exigencies of life, that they are more often influenced in their judgments by feelings of affection or hostility—all these would be amply accounted for by the modification in the formation of their super-ego which we have inferred above. We must not allow ourselves to be deflected from such conclusions by the denials of the feminists, who are anxious to force us to regard the two sexes as completely equal in position and worth; but we shall, of course, willingly agree that the majority of men are also far behind the masculine ideal and

that all human individuals, as a result of their bisexual disposition and of cross-inheritance, combine in themselves both masculine and feminine characteristics, so that pure masculinity and femininity remain theoretical constructions of uncertain content" ([1925b] 1995, 257).

6. Anna Freud, of Freud's children the only one who became a psychoanalyst, tended to her father during his almost thirty surgeries for mouth cancer. He had many prostheses as well as wounds that needed to be cleaned out daily. She lived with Freud in London after they fled Vienna because of World War II. See Young-Breuhl (1994).

7. Freud famously struggled with his women patients throughout his life, something that we can see best in his one female case from 1905, *Fragment of an Analysis of a Case of Hysteria*, where he invents the concept of transference and countertransference in order to explain his blindness to the patient's homosexual desire as well as her rage against Freud. What is unresolved in Freud's countertransference we certainly inherit as a discipline.

8. Ego psychology was theorized by Anna Freud and then taken up by analysts in America, notably Heinz Hartmann, Ernst Kris, and Rudolph Lowenstein. Distinct in tone, theory, and technique is the British tradition following the work of Melanie Klein. Both theories seek a solution to the conundrums of guilt, aggression, and symptom formation as linked to the relationship between the ego and superego. For the ego psychologists, a healthier defense structure created by analyzing "infantile" wishes would help a patient adapt to "reality." For the Kleinians, aggressive fantasies need to be brought to the surface of a treatment to help bring patients closer to their depressive feelings and wishes for reparation, lessening the need for schizoid and manic defenses against internal and external "reality."

9. See Foucault's *Discipline and Punish* (1975), where the eighteenth-century image of a perfect penal institution in which every inmate can be watched by a single observer becomes the model of modern surveillance and disciplinary society. In a way, this is already close to how Freud described the superego, the "over-I," which knows everything both conscious and unconscious. You don't even need to think about committing a transgressive act—to wish it or think it is enough for punishment.

10. The superego keeps a vigilant watch over the body's states of excitement, and these two can be seen as engaged in an interminable standoff in the same way that morality, religious and secular, has always been directed at the body, especially women's bodies. Of course, this is an important thread in Foucault's work on religious and governmental institutions and their discipline of the body. Here we might link Foucault and Lacan, despite their mutual suspicions.

11. See Arnaud (2015) and Gherovici (2003) for a history of hysteria.

12. In Freud's paper "Instincts and their Vicissitudes," he writes, "If now we apply ourselves to considering mental life from a *biological* point of view, an 'instinct' appears to us as a concept on the frontier between the mental and the somatic, as the psychical representative of the stimuli originating from within the organism and reaching the mind, as a measure of the demand made upon the mind for work in consequence of its connection with the body" ([1915] 1995, 121–22).

13. Freud's "Some Character Types Met with in Psychoanalytic Work" has a section titled "Criminals from a Sense of Guilt" ([1916] 1995), where he says that paradoxically guilt is present before misdeeds and that the criminal seeks a crime to fit his guilt and need for punishment.

II. MUSIC OF THE FUTURE

1. Freud's called his early unpublished work on the etiology of neuroses his *neurotica*—seemingly a joke about his "neurotic" desire for a comprehensive system of diagnosis. It was begun in concert with his self-analysis transforming into a desire to write about dreams—common to us all—rather than psychopathology.

III. FATHER CAN'T YOU SEE

1. The following account of a psychotic patient is paraphrased from a long transcript of a dialogue between this patient and Lacan, published in 1980 in English in *Returning to Freud: Clinical Psychoanalysis in the School of Lacan* (Lacan 1980).

IV. NEVER THE RIGHT MAN

1. Monique David-Ménard and Isabelle Alfandary in many works on hysteria and conversion have argued extensively that Freud needed to keep the leap from psyche to soma in conversion as an undefined gap without a direct linguistic connection. Conversion used old pathways already innervated rather than creating new ones on the basis of a linguistic representation. See David-Ménard (1989).
2. This is seen most clearly in Freud and Breuer's ([1895] 1995) *Studies in Hysteria*.
3. Lacan in "L'étourdit" (1972a, b) says that the love of women is always to love what remains Other.
4. See chapter 10 regarding the "monstrous" "ethical" relation of the psychoanlayst to the drive. One might call this a kind of identification or accomodation of drive life, what is here being pointed to by the notion of remorselessness and sublimation.

V. I AM NOT A MUSE

1. Freud, in discussing the various regimes of seeking pleasure and avoiding unpleasure, says the following about love: "I am, of course, speaking of the way of life which makes love the centre of everything, which looks for all satisfaction in loving and being loved. A psychical attitude of this sort comes naturally enough to all of us; one of the forms in which love manifests itself—sexual love—has given us our most

intense experience of an overwhelming sensation of pleasure and has thus furnished us with a pattern for our search for happiness. What is more natural than that we should persist in looking for happiness along the path on which we first encountered it? The weak side of this technique of living is easy to see; otherwise no human being would have thought of abandoning this path to happiness for any other. It is that we are never so defenceless against suffering as when we love, never so helplessly unhappy as when we have lost our loved object or its love. But this does not dispose of the technique of living based on the value of love as a means to happiness" ([1930] 1995, 82).

VI. HYSTERICAL RUINOLOGY

1. Agamben relies on a psychoanalytic concept of trauma where a system is overwhelmed from the outside by something too real—forever trying to catch up to this moment. Freud in his 1920 work *Beyond the Pleasure Principle* pointed to the repetition of the traumatic moment in war neuroses, in dreams, and in constant anxiety, where every moment is somehow judged on the basis of the prior trauma—am I in danger again, or am I not? Is this the same terror, or am I safe? Agamben takes this concept and applies it to the contemporary world, which he says lives in a constant state of crises, not the least of which is seen in the perpetual war on terror.
2. "Bare life" is a concept used by Agamben to denote when someone's life has been reduced to biology because their political or subjective existence has been negated by those who have the power to decide who and who isn't given a voice even while their lives remain bound to the regulations of governmental power.
3. Lacan can be seen as venerating the figure of the saint, especially in *On Feminine Sexuality, The Limits of Love and Knowledge (Encore), Book XX* (1999). His position in "L'étourdit" seems significantly more skeptical than his infamous praise of Saint Teresa, or even of Bataille as a male mystic, in Seminar XX.

VII. *COITUS INTERRUPTUS*

1. *Coitus interruptus* is a fascinating example of how Freud's theory of the symptom can be more intersubjective than intrasubjective. Many theorists saw Freud as too centered on the individual, outside of his or her relations with others, and read an intersubjective or relational framework back into his thinking. Here, with anxiety—a concept that tends toward a reading of an "inner," isolated experience—we have Freud rendering anxiety through an intersubjective dynamic, the effect of a sexual encounter.
2. For more, see "Draft E—How Anxiety Originates" (in Freud 1985). In particular, Freud begins to attempt to categorize the effects of sexual practices on anxiety in the sexes:

> With this aim in view, I brought together the cases in which I found anxiety arising from a sexual cause. They seemed at first to be quite heterogeneous:

(1) Anxiety in *virginal* people (sexual observations and in formation, foreshadowings of sexual life); confirmed by numerous instances of both sexes, predominantly female. Not infrequently there is a hint at an intermediate link—a sensation like an erection arising in the genitals. (2) Anxiety in *intentionally abstinent* people, *prudes* (a type of neuropath), men and women characterized by pedantry and a feeling for cleanliness, who regard everything sexual as horrible. The same people tend to work their anxiety over into phobias, obsessional actions, *folie du doute*. (3) Anxiety of *necessarily abstinent* people, women who are neglected by their husbands or are not satisfied on account of lack of potency. This form of anxiety neurosis can certainly be acquired, and, owing to subsidiary circumstances, is often combined with neurasthenia. (4) Anxiety of women living with coitus interruptus, or, what is similar, of women whose husbands suffer from ejaculatio praecox—of people, therefore, in whom physical stimulation is not satisfied. (5) Anxiety of men practicing coitus interruptus, even more of men who excite themselves in various ways and do not employ their erection for coitus. (6) Anxiety of men *who go beyond their desire or strength*, older people whose potency is diminishing, but who nevertheless forcibly bring about coitus. (7) Anxiety of men who abstain on occasion: of youngish men who have married older women, by whom they are in fact disgusted, or of *neurasthenics* who have been diverted from masturbation by intellectual occupation without making up for it by coitus, or of men whose potency is beginning to grow weak and who abstain in marriage on account of sensations *post coitum*. In the remaining cases the connection between the anxiety and sexual life was not obvious. (It could be established theoretically.)

How are all these separate cases to be brought together? What recurs in them most frequently is abstinence. Taught by the fact that even anaesthetic women are subject to anxiety after *coitus interruptus*, one is inclined to say that it is a question of a physical accumulation of excitation—that is, *an accumulation of physical sexual tension*. The accumulation is the consequence of discharge being prevented. Thus anxiety neurosis is a neurosis of damming-up, like hysteria; hence their similarity. And since no anxiety at all is contained in what is accumulated, the position is expressed by saying that *anxiety* has arisen by *transformation* out of the accumulated sexual tension.

(79–80)

3. Freud was admiring and critical of Otto Rank's theory of birth trauma. In a letter to Karl Abraham from February 15, 1924, he writes: "Here Rank differs from me. He refuses to go into phylogenesis and lets the anxiety, which opposes incest, directly repeat the birth anxiety, so that, he says, the neurotic regression into oneself is inhibited by the nature of the birth process. This birth anxiety, he says, is transferred to the father, but he is only a pretext for it. Basically the attitude to the mother's body or genital is assumed to be *a priori* an ambivalent one. This the contradiction. I find it

very difficult to decide here, nor do I see how one can easily succeed from experience, for in analysis we shall always come upon the father as the bearer of the prohibition. But that is naturally no argument. I must for the time being leave the question open. I can bring forward as a counter-argument also that it is not in the nature of an instinct to be associatively inhibited, as here the instinct to return to the mother would be by association with the fright of birth. Actually every instinct as a drive to re-establish a former state presupposes a trauma as the cause of the change, and so there could be no other than ambivalent instincts, i.e. instincts accompanied by anxiety" (Freud 2002, 481–482).

4. While Freud theorized about the importance of exhibitionism and scopophilia in the *Three Essays on the Theory of Sexuality* ([1905c] 1995), Lacan furthers this, making the gaze one of the objects of the drive. The gaze can be an important organizer of the drive in a way that props up a subject through a fantasized gaze, either their own or the watching Other.

VIII. THREE VISIONS OF PSYCHOANALYSIS

1. Bachelard's work calls for a psychoanalytic critique of science and the philosophy of science. Important to Bachelard is that we see the discontinuous nature of scientific inquiry, which tends to need to counter human illusions, especially narcissistic illusions that influence their understanding. The scientific object for him is complex; built up through theory, error, and experimentation; and never static. In his work with the notion of fire, Bachelard hopes to find a more primordial object before the sedimentations of narcissism, moral order, and the presumptions of positivist science.

2. Foucault was notoriously antipsychoanalytic. He saw psychoanalysis as a form of discipline and knowledge too close to psychiatry and other forms of mental "hygiene." Nevertheless, I find in this early work on literature and madness a credence given to the project of psychoanalysis as if it is the last bulwark against the attempt by civilization to tame and eradicate madness. Because this work is tied to questions of language, and language that attempts to preserve itself through madness, it seems fitting for him to have a more positive inclination toward the psychoanalytic project. More than this, Foucault's work on what language might look like if it succeeded in eradicating madness and what we can learn from the history of literature as a mad project seems deeply prophetic to me of postmodern, post-truth currents, which seem even more disciplinary than liberating—at least right now. Again, I am pointing to some last threshold in the twin projects of literature and psychoanalysis as tied to a question of madness. Foucault would turn against much of his early work, seeing neither literature nor psychoanalysis as able to point toward a more ethical life. And while in some measure I think he is right and that the distinctions ought to be considered carefully, in this section I want to point to what he saw in literature and psychoanalysis that might be carried forward and that anticipates a reinvigoration of

the question of psychosis for psychoanalytic work, especially as a means of countering the idealization of the hallmarks of neurosis from reflexive interiority to autonomy, etc.

IX. HOW TO SPLINTER / HOW TO BURN

1. Both the first written-about psychoanalytic case, Anna O., as well as Dora, suffered from a hysterical pregnancy that seemed to crown the efforts of treatment. While the patients had many conversion symptoms, the pains associated with a phantom pregnancy seem to speak to something important about the question of conversion and its ties to sexuality, the body, and the transference to the analyst.
2. Lacan often characterized hysteria as the choice of an unsatisfied desire against *jouissance* or enjoyment. The hysteric would rather prop herself up as not getting what she wants from the other because there is a fear of satisfaction, especially in its sexual dimension. Here I am trying to add some subtlety—perhaps there is a distaste for the way satisfaction is offered up by contemporary society, and she seeks to speak to the delicacy of the relationship between desire and enjoyment, to tie the two together in a new way.

X. FORGED IN STONES

1. In Gaddis, the main argument of the novel centers on a question of original sin that cannot be escaped. Writing during the backlash against 1950s American morality, Gaddis is dubious about that liberatory project.
2. One of the few films made of Lacan is one of a 1969 lecture he gave in Leuven, where he is famously interrupted by a situationist protestor. In the beginning of the talk, before the protestor, he speaks about his patient's dream and the importance of death in the life of a subject.

REFERENCES

Agamben, Giorgio. 1993. *The Coming Community*. Trans. Michael Hardt. Minneapolis: University of Minnesota Press.
——. 1995. *Homo Sacer: Sovereign Power and Bare Life*. Trans. D. Heller-Roazen. Stanford, CA: Stanford University Press.
——. 2005. *State of Exception*. Trans. K Atell. Chicago: University of Chicago Press.
——. 2009. *Signature of All Things: On Method*. Trans. L D'Isanto. New York: Zone.
——. 2011. *The Kingdom and the Glory*. Trans. Lorenzo Chiesa and Matteo Mandarini. Stanford, CA: University Press.
——. 2013. *The Highest Poverty: Monastic Rules and Form-of-Life*. Trans. A. Kotsko. Stanford, CA: Stanford University Press.
——. 2015. *Pilate and Jesus*. Trans. A. Kotsko. Stanford, CA: Stanford University Press.
American Psychiatric Association. 2013. *Diagnostic and Statistical Manual of Mental Disorders: DSM-V*. Arlington, VA: American Psychiatric Publishing.
Aristophanes. 1962. *The Clouds*. Trans. W. Arrowsmith. New York: Mentor.
Arnaud, Sabine. 2015. *On Hysteria: The Invention of a Medical Category*. Chicago: University of Chicago Press.
Bachelard, Gaston. 1964. *The Psychoanalysis of Fire*. Trans. A. C. M. Ross. Boston: Beacon.
Benjamin, Walter. 2008. *The Work of Art in the Age of Mechanical Reproducibility and Other Writings on Media*. Ed. B. Doherty and T. Levin. Cambridge, MA: Belknap.
Blanchot, Maurice. 1988. *The Unavowable Community*. Trans. Pierre Joris. Barrytown, NY: Station Hill.
——. 1995. *The Work of Fire*. Trans. C. Mandell. Stanford, CA: Stanford University Press.
Büchner, Georg. 1994. *Danton's Death*. In *Complete Plays, Lenz, and Other Writings*. New York: Penguin.
Celan, Paul. 2011. *The Meridian: Final Version—Drafts—Materials*. Trans. Bernhard Boschenstein. Stanford, CA: Stanford University Press.

Claudel, Paul. 1945. *Three Plays: The Hostage, Crusts, The Humiliation of the Father*. Trans. J. Heard. Boston: John. W. Luce.
David-Ménard, Monique. 1989. *Hysteria from Freud to Lacan: Body and Language in Psychoanalysis*. Trans. C. Porter. Ithaca, NY: Cornell University Press.
Ferenczi, Sándor. 1949. "Confusion of the Tongues Between the Adults and the Child: The Language of Tenderness and of Passion." *International Journal of Psycho-Analysis* 30:225–30.
Fink, Bruce. 2013. *Against Understanding: Commentary and Critique in a Lacanian Key*. 2 vols. New York: Routledge.
Foucault, Michel. 1975. *Discipline and Punish: The Birth of the Prison*. New York: Vintage.
——. 1977. "Nietzsche, Genealogy, History." In *Language, Counter-Memory, Practice: Selected Essays and Interviews*, ed. D. Bouchard. Ithaca, NY: Cornell University Press.
——. 1993. Preface to *Dream and Existence*, by Michel Foucault and Ludwig Binswanger, ed. Keith Hoeller. Atlantic Highlands, NJ: Humanities Press.
——. 1995. "Madness, the Absence of Work." *Critical Inquiry* 21 (2): 290–298.
——. 2006. *Maurice Blanchot: The Thought from Outside*. Trans. J. Mehlman. New York: Zone.
——. 2015. *Language, Madness, and Desire: On Literature*. Trans. R. Bononno. Minneapolis: University of Minnesota Press.
Freud, Sigmund. (1894) 1995. "The Neuro-psychoses of Defence." In *The Standard Edition of the Complete Psychological Works of Sigmund Freud*, 3:43–61.
——. (1895) 1995. "Project for a Scientific Psychology." In *The Standard Edition of the Complete Psychological Works of Sigmund Freud*, 1:283–397.
——. (1896) 1995. "The Aetiology of Hysteria." In *The Standard Edition of the Complete Psychological Works of Sigmund Freud*, 3:189–221.
——. (1899) 1995. "Screen Memories." In *The Standard Edition of the Complete Psychological Works of Sigmund Freud*, 3:301–22.
——. (1900) 1995. *The Interpretation of Dreams*. In *The Standard Edition of the Complete Psychological Works of Sigmund Freud*, vols. 4–5.
——. (1905a) 1995. "Fragment of an Analysis of a Case of Hysteria." In *The Standard Edition of the Complete Psychological Works of Sigmund Freud*, 7:1–122.
——. (1905b) 1995. *Jokes and Their Relation to the Unconscious*. In *The Standard Edition of the Complete Psychological Works of Sigmund Freud*, vol. 8.
——. (1905c) 1995. *Three Essays on the Theory of Sexuality*. In *The Standard Edition of the Complete Psychological Works of Sigmund Freud*, 7:125–245.
——. (1910) 1995. "A Special Type of Choice of Object Made by Men." In *The Standard Edition of the Complete Psychological Works of Sigmund Freud*, 11:165–75.
——. (1912) 1995. "The Universal Tendency Towards Debasement in the Sphere of Love." In *The Standard Edition of the Complete Psychological Works of Sigmund Freud*, 11:179–90.
——. (1913a) 1995. "The Theme of Three Caskets." In *The Standard Edition of the Complete Psychological Works of Sigmund Freud*, 12:289–302.
——. (1913b) 1995. *Totem and Taboo*. In *The Standard Edition of the Complete Psychological Works of Sigmund Freud*, 13:1–161.

———. (1914) 1995. "On Narcissism: An Introduction." In *The Standard Edition of the Complete Psychological Works of Sigmund Freud*, 14:67–102.

———. (1915) 1995. "Instincts and Their Vicissitudes." In *The Standard Edition of the Complete Psychological Works of Sigmund Freud*, 14:109–40.

———. (1916) 1995. "Criminals from a Sense of Guilt." In "Some Character Types Met with in Psycho-Analytic Work." In *The Standard Edition of the Complete Psychological Works of Sigmund Freud*, 14:309–33.

———. (1917a) 1995. "Mourning and Melancholia." In *The Standard Edition of the Complete Psychological Works of Sigmund Freud*, 14:239–58.

———. (1917b) 1995. "Introductory Lectures on Psychoanalysis." In *The Standard Edition of the Complete Psychological Works of Sigmund Freud*, 16:243–456.

———. (1918) 1995. "The Taboo on Virginity." In *The Standard Edition of the Complete Psychological Works of Sigmund Freud*, 11:191–208.

———. (1921) 1995. *Group Psychology and the Analysis of the Ego*. In *The Standard Edition of the Complete Psychological Works of Sigmund Freud*, 18:67–143.

———. (1925a) 1995. "Negation." In *The Standard Edition of the Complete Psychological Works of Sigmund Freud*, 19:235–239.

———. (1925b) 1995. "Some Psychical Consequences of the Anatomical Distinction Between the Sexes." In *The Standard Edition of the Complete Psychological Works of Sigmund Freud*, 19:243–58.

———. (1926) 1995. *Inhibitions, Symptoms, and Anxiety*. In *The Standard Edition of the Complete Psychological Works of Sigmund Freud*, 20:77–174.

———. (1930) 1995. *Civilization and Its Discontents*. In *The Standard Edition of the Complete Psychological Works of Sigmund Freud*, 21:59–145.

———. (1931) 1995. "Female Sexuality." In *The Standard Edition of the Complete Psychological Works of Sigmund Freud*, 21:221–43.

———. (1938) 1995. "Findings, Ideas, Problems." In *The Standard Edition of the Complete Psychological Works of Sigmund Freud*, 23:299–300.

———. 1985. *The Complete Letters of Sigmund Freud to Wilhelm Fleiss*. Trans. J. Masson. Cambridge, MA: Harvard University Press.

———. 1995. *The Standard Edition of the Complete Psychological Works of Sigmund Freud*. Trans. and ed. James Strachey. 24 vols. London: Hogarth.

———. 2002. *The Complete Correspondence of Sigmund Freud and Karl Abraham, 1907–1925*. Ed. E. Falzender. New York: Routledge.

Freud, Sigmund, and Josef Breuer. (1893) 1995. "On the Psychical Mechanism of Hysterical Phenomena." In *Studies in Hysteria*. In *The Standard Edition of the Complete Psychological Works of Sigmund Freud*, 2:1–17.

———. (1895) 1995. *Studies in Hysteria*. In *The Standard Edition of the Complete Psychological Works of Sigmund Freud*, 2:1–319.

Gaddis, William. 1993. *The Recognitions*. New York: Penguin.

Gherovici, Patricia. 2003. *The Puerto Rican Syndrome*. New York: Other Press.

Gitelson, Maxwell. 1954. "Therapeutic Problems in the Analysis of the 'Normal' Candidate." *International Journal of Psychoanalysis* 35:174–183.

Grosskurth, Phyllis. 1991. *The Secret Ring: Freud's Inner Circle and the Politics of Psychoanalysis*. Reading, MA: Addison-Wesley.
Heiddeger, Martin. 1971. "Building, Dwelling, Thinking." In *Poetry, Language, Thought*, trans. A. Hofstadter. New York: Harper & Row.
Jacoby, Russel. 1996. *Social Amnesia: A Critique of Contemporary Psychology*. New York: Routledge.
James, William. (1902) 1982. *The Varieties of Religious Experience: A Study in Human Nature*. New York: Penguin.
Kantorowicz, Ernst. 1957. *The King's Two Bodies*. Princeton, NJ: Princeton University Press.
Knight, R. P. 1953. "The Present Status of Organized Psychoanalysis in the United States." *Journal of the American Psychoanalytic Association* 1 (2): 197–221.
Lacan, Jacques. 1966–1967. *The Logic of Fantasy*. Jacques Lacan in Ireland Seminars. http://www.lacaninireland.com/web/wp-content/uploads/2010/06/14-Logic-of-Phantasy-Complete.pdf.
———. 1967–1968. *The Psychoanalytic Act*. Jacques Lacan in Ireland Seminars. http://www.lacaninireland.com/web/wp-content/uploads/2010/06/Book-15-The-Psychoanalytical-Act.pdf.
———. 1970–1971. *On a Discourse That Might Not Be a Semblance*. Jacques Lacan in Ireland Seminars. http://www.lacaninireland.com/web/wp-content/uploads/2010/06/Book-18-On-a-discourse-that-might-not-be-a-semblance.pdf.
———. 1971–1972. *The Knowledge of the Psychoanalyst*. Jacques Lacan in Ireland Seminars. http://www.lacaninireland.com/web/wp-content/uploads/2010/06/Book-19a-The-Knowledge-of-the-Psychoanalyst-1971-1972.pdf.
———. 1972a. "L'étourdit (1972)." Jacques Lacan in Ireland Ecrits. http://www.lacaninireland.com/web/wp-content/uploads/2010/06/JL-etourdit-CG-Trans-Letter-41.pdf.
———. 1972b. "L'étourdit: Turn Two." Jacques Lacan in Ireland Ecrits. http://www.lacaninireland.com/web/wp-content/uploads/2010/06/etourdit-Second-turn-Final-Version4.pdf.
———. (1973) 1990. *Television*. Trans. D. Hollier, R. Krauss, and A. Michelson. New York: Norton.
———. 1977. "Propos sur l'hysterie." *Quarto* 2:5–10.
———. 1980. "A Lacanian Psychosis." In *Returning to Freud: Clinical Psychoanalysis in the School of Lacan*, ed. S. Schneiderman. New Haven, CT: Yale University Press.
———. 1981. *Seminar: Book XI: The Four Fundamental Concepts of Psychoanalysis*. Trans. A. Sheridan. New York: Norton.
———. 1991. *Seminar: Book II: The Ego in Freud's Theory and in the Technique of Psychoanalysis, 1954–1955*. Trans. A. Sheridan. New York: Norton.
———. 1997. *The Seminar of Jacques Lacan: The Ethics of Psychoanalysis (Book VII)*. Ed. J.-A. Miller. New York: Norton.
———. 1999. *On Feminine Sexuality, The Limits of Love and Knowledge (Encore), Book XX*. Trans. B. Fink. New York: Norton.
———. 2006. *Écrits: The First Complete Edition in English*. Trans. B. Fink. New York: Norton.
———. 2014. *Anxiety. The Seminar of Jacques Lacan, Book X*. Trans. A. R. Price. Cambridge: Polity.

———. 2016. *Transference. The Seminar of Jacques Lacan, Book VIII*. Trans. B. Fink. London: Polity.
———. 2017. *The Sinthome. The Seminar of Jacques Lacan, Book XXIII*. Ed. J.-A. Miller. London: Polity.
Leclaire, Serge. 1998. *Psychoanalyzing: On the Order of the Unconscious and the Practice of the Letter*. Trans. P. Kamuf. Stanford, CA: Stanford University Press.
———. 2012. "The Analyst in His Place." In *Concept and Form: Key Texts from* Cahiers pour l'Analyse, ed. P. Hallward and K. Peden, 1:103–6. New York: Verso.
Lispector, Clarice. 2012a. *Near to the Wild Heart*. Trans. A. Entrekin. New York: New Directions.
———. 2012b. *The Passion According to GH*. Trans. I. Novey. New York: New Directions.
Melville, Herman. (1892) 1996. *Pierre; or, The Ambiguities*. New York: Penguin.
Michaux, Henri. 2016. *Life in the Folds*. Trans. D. Jackson. Cambridge: Wakefield.
Miller, Jacques-Alain. 2015. "The Unconscious and the Speaking Body." In *The Speaking Body: On the Unconscious in the Twenty-First Century*. Scilicet: NLS Publication.
Nancy, Jean-Luc. 1991. *The Inoperative Community*. Minneapolis: University of Minnesota Press.
———. 2008. *Corpus*. Trans. R. Rand. New York: Fordham University Press.
Nietzsche, Friedrich. 1901. *The Will to Power*. Trans. W. Kaufman. New York: Vintage.
Nock, A. D. 1933. *Conversion: The Old and New in Religion from Alexander the Great to Hippo*. Baltimore, MD: John Hopkins University Press.
Reik, Theodore. 1949. *Listening with the Third Ear: The Inner Experience of a Psychoanalyst*. New York: Farrar, Straus and Giroux.
Rieff, Phillip. 1959. *Freud: The Mind of the Moralist*. Chicago: University of Chicago Press.
———. 1966. *The Triumph of the Therapeutic*. New York: Harper & Row.
Robertson, Lisa. 2005. *Magenta Soul Whip*. Toronto: Coach House.
———. 2006. *The Men: A Lyric Book*. Toronto: Book Thug.
Young-Breuhl, Elisabeth. 1994. *Anna Freud: A Biography*. New York: Norton.

INDEX

abjection, 149–151, 206, 208–210, 212, 218
accident, 210–214, 222, 238–239
affect, 11, 62–63, 74–77, 152, 163, 167, 184, 220–222; bodily movement and, 99–100, 110, 119, 132–133, 223, 265–266; clinical case histories and, 126; conversion and, 11, 75–77, 211, 272; fears and, 105–106, 116, 159, 164, 207, 217, 220–221; Freud on, 62–63, 74; language and, 90, 197, 206–208, 231, 256
affirmation, 139, 141–142, 145; and feminine desire, 169–170, 174, 178, 206–208, 210, 279, 282
Agamben, Giorgio: on angels, 145; on dreams, 91–92; on irreparability, 34, 37, 147; on libidinal economy, 26- 27, 69, 138; on messianism, 139; on Pilate and Jesus, 146–147; political theology, 136–138; temporality, 54; trauma 136–137, 147
Agamben, Giorgio, works of: *The Highest Poverty: Monastic Rules and Form-of-Life* (2013), 139; *Homo Sacer: Sovereign Power and Bare Life* (1995), 138; *The Kingdom and the Glory* (2011), 138, 142; "Philosophical Archaeology" (2009), 139; *The Signature of All Things* (2009), 137
anesthesia, 81, 83, 103, 271
anxiety, 5, 6, 55–56, 66, 68, 156, 168, 177, 216, 266, 271; and castration, 66, 164–165, 168, 218; and excitation, 5–7; and hysteria, 13, 67–68,75; and sexuality, 157, 165, 288
asocial, 111–114
association, 77, 81, 83, 109, 204, 260, 277, 280, 289; as free association, 19, 197, 201, 213
attachment, 99, 163–164, 173, 278
autonomy, 22–24, 139, 146, 165, 284n2

Bachelard, Gaston: psychoanalysis of fire, 181–185
Benjamin, Walter: reproducibility of aesthetic object, 210–211, 214
biopolitics, 136–138. *See also* Agamben, Giorgio; Foucault, Michel
body, 52–52, 59, 72–73, 84, 134, 145, 154, 156, 173, 177, 190–191, 204, 208, 216–217; appendix, 275, 281–282; in pieces (*corps morsele*), 55, 75–77, 85, 191, 216, 224, 260; and bodily refusal, 13, 37, 42, 43, 47, 71, 108–109, 113, 131, 223, 266, 276; and communication, 36, 40, 51–52, 58–60, 88, 122, 157, 177, 186, 188, 206, 220–221; and depression, 48, 82–83, 113, 209; and language 14–15, 50–51, 55, 88, 99, 109, 187, 190, 194, 220, 223; and mnemic symbol, 73–74, 76; psyche and soma, 11, 45, 62–63, 78, 80, 84, 109, 115, 159, 167, 223–224; and regulatory power, 31, 136; and sexuality, 21, 77, 191, 272

Celan, Paul: "Meridian Speech" (1960), 117, 121–122
countertransference, 18, 38, 124, 168, 234, 285n7
cure, 4, 8, 34–35, 39, 63, 76, 85, 114–115, 154, 164, 177, 193, 214, 228–229, 235, 238; as conversion of analyst, 35, 221–223, 226, 272; crooked cure, 6, 112, 115; and Eastern medicine, 1, 5, 275–276; as embodiment, 59, 228–229; and pharmacological intervention, 1, 5; as *pharmakon*, 132–133, 233

death drive, 37, 44, 118, 161, 218–219, 241, 226, 241
diagnosis, 26, 44, 67–68, 107, 118, 122; of culture, 157
difference, 106, 173, 186, 189, 209, 212–214, 225–226, 232, 234, 267; sexual, 90, 159, 207, 218
disappearance, 8, 27, 68, 112, 118–121, 130, 132, 145, 148, 194, 212, 225, 247–248, 260, 266
displacement, 70, 91, 122, 143–144, 163, 235, 257, 270; and dispossession, 216
dreams, 30, 68, 89–92, 94, 98, 183, 191, 211–213, 225, 228–231, 234, 267–268, 272, 277–278, 281
dreams, Freud's: burning child, 93–95; of father's death, 99; Irma injection, 93–95, 124, 150
drive, 14, 43, 120, 128, 142–143, 156–157, 166, 216, 221, 223–227, 230–233, 235, 264
discontent, 48, 64–66, 80, 83, 85, 114, 163, 193, 262, 275
dissociation, 126, 241
Duras, Marguerite, 248

economy of desire, 80–81, 138, 142–145, 162, 167, 221–222, 226, 232, 234, 259–260, 270; and conversion, 219, 244
ego, 70–71, 73–74, 78, 83, 104, 110, 113–114, 161–163, 187, 257
ego-ideal, 110, 113–114, 218, 243, 255–256, 260, 264
ego psychology, 22, 41, 216, 255, 285n8

Empedocles Complex, 182–183. *See also* Bachelard, Gaston
end of analysis, 66, 152, 154, 168, 204, 221, 234, 242–243, 245, 249, 280; and closure, 37, 98–100, 143, 232
envy, 34, 55, 170; penis envy, 66, 169, 174, 217
ethics, 139, 144, 216, 233, 243
exteriority, 5, 32, 40, 58, 65, 71, 84, 97, 156–157, 162, 165, 167–168, 172, 174, 177, 181, 187, 192, 200, 207, 220, 271

failure, 103, 210, 238, 260; and psychoanalysis, 149, 201, 222, 234; and sexual relations, 103, 106, 156, 166, 168
family, 47, 111, 123, 161, 182–183, 206–210, 213, 232, 240, 250, 258, 260–262, 268–271, 277–279
femininity, 14, 25, 26, 62–63, 66, 111, 133, 168–169, 174–175, 204–205, 238, 279; blood/menstruation, 206–207, 278; and enjoyment, 41, 128, 169–173, 175, 210, 280–282; and female bodies, 47, 205–206, 217, 278; and frigidity, 103, 107, 168; and Madonna/whore complex, 102; and resistance, 104, 107–108, 160; and sexual bondage, 104, 107–108, 115; and taboo, 106, 108; and virginity, 102, 104–105, 108, 118, 156, 262
Ferenczi, Sándor, 283n1
flesh, 51, 54, 59, 153, 208, 211–213, 230
Foucault, Michel: language and exteriorization, 181, 195, 197; "Madness, the Absence of Work" (1995), 32–33; "Nietzsche, Genealogy, History" (1977), 140; psychoanalysis of madness, 193–195, 197–200
fragmentation, 68–69, 75, 133, 138, 149, 156, 216, 224, 277
Freud, Anna, 41, 239–241, 244, 251, 285n6, 285n8
Freud, Sigmund: and Krafft-Ebing, 104; letters to Fliess, 53, 67, 72, 78, 103, 158, 160, 234; on limit concepts, 216; and misogyny, 103, 107; and pleasure principle, 78, 82, 156, 242–243
Freud, Sigmund, case histories: Anna O., 38, 72, 122; Little Hans, 59; Dora, 59, 66,

69, 103, 123, 261, 276–281; Emmy von N., 122; Wolf Man, 59; Female homosexual, 123; Case of paranoia, 123; Rat Man, 259–261

Freud, Sigmund, works: "The Aetiology of Hysteria" (1896), 7; "Analysis Terminable and Interminable" (1937), 170, 242; "A Child Is Being Beaten" (1919), 256–257; *Civilization and Its Discontents* (1930), 37, 64, 82, 118, 123, 143, 161, 193; "A Disturbance of Memory on the Acropolis" (1935), 238–241, 269; *Group Psychology and the Analysis of the Ego* (1921), 103, 110, 113, 160; *Inhibitions, Symptoms, and Anxiety* (1926), 70, 72, 164, 280; *The Interpretation of Dreams* (1900), 68, 85, 92–93, 100, 159, 254, 281 (*see also* self-analysis); "Jokes and Their Relation to the Unconscious" (1905), 257; "Mourning and Melancholia" (1917), 102; "On Narcissism" (1914), 102; "The Neuro-psychoses of Defense" (1894), 68; *Psychopathology of Everyday Life* (1901), 238; "Project for a Scientific Psychology" (1895), 142; "Screen Memories" (1899), 261; "Some Psychical Consequences of the Anatomical Distinction Between the Sexes" (1925), 218; "A Special Type of Choice of Object Made by Men" (1910), 102; *Studies in Hysteria* (1895), 62–67, 73, 109; "The Subtleties of a Faulty Action" (1935), 238; "The Taboo on Virginity" (1918), 102, 110, 113; "The Theme of the Three Caskets" (1913), 241; *Three Essays on the Theory of Sexuality*, 59, 187, 213–214; *Totem and Taboo* (1913), 102, 112; "The Universal Tendency Towards Debasement in the Sphere of Love" (1912), 102

future, 10, 16, 26, 32, 35–36, 42, 46, 53–54, 88, 90, 97, 105, 111, 126, 132–134, 137, 141, 144, 181, 193, 216, 251, 255, 258. *See also* temporality

Gaddis, William, 227–228, 290n1
gaze, 127–128, 152, 164, 170–173, 177–178
Gide, André, 248
gift, 238–244

Gitelson, Maxwell: "Therapeutic Problems in the Analysis of the 'Normal' Candidate" (1954), 264–265. *See also* training analysis

glory, 142, 145

group psychology, 6, 40, 102, 106, 110–112; and collective narrative, 214

guilt, 2, 14, 16, 18, 38–40, 47–48, 114–116, 126, 150, 153, 161, 166, 209, 225, 241, 243, 270, 285n8, 286n13

hallucination, 67–68, 73, 80, 85, 96, 114, 262. *See also* nightmare

Heidegger, Martin, 233

humor, 120, 229, 230, 232, 266, 272; joke, 167, 185, 205, 227, 230, 232, 257–258, 272, 286

hysteria, 12, 27, 40, 53, 66–68, 84, 112, 114, 118, 120, 122, 165, 188–189, 212, 228, 276; and angels, 146; architecture of, 73, 75–76, 139, 164, 188; and art, 112, 212; in contemporary culture, 119, 122; hysterical amnesia, 72, 75, 217, 219, 228; and language, 69–70, 149, 219; and laughter, 120, 134, 146, 230; and phantom limb, 58, 165 (*see also* illness: psychosomatic); and the symptom, 71, 83, 94, 188, 207, 229, 278–280

idealization, 175, 185, 201, 218, 226, 234, 255, 267, 290n2

identification, 53, 113–114, 125, 127, 131, 134, 164, 204, 216–217, 265, 279

illness, 5, 11, 25, 48, 64–65, 143, 160, 241, 272; appendicitis, 275–281; hypochondria, 11–13, 47, 158; psychosomatic, 11–13, 44, 73, 77, 109. *See also* hysteria: and the symptom

imaginary, 234, 255–256, 266

impossibility, 48, 50, 146, 149, 152–153, 199, 210, 219, 226; and bodily processes, 156; and incommensurability, 147; and psychoanalytic profession, 37, 42, 46, 54, 59, 95, 148, 151, 216, 233, 235, 251, 272; and the real, 92, 114, 223, 225

indeterminacy, 6, 10, 43, 157, 165–167, 174, 177–178, 190, 193, 258, 264, 280

inhibition, 78, 82, 102–103, 110, 160, 183, 217

interiority, 5, 32, 40, 58, 65, 71, 80, 84, 97, 156–157, 162, 168, 176–177, 181, 184, 194, 200, 207, 214
interpretation, 137, 143, 148, 189, 204, 222, 238, 251, 259, 265, 270
interruption, 156–157, 166–167, 175, 239
intimacy, 7, 34, 54, 74, 219, 279

James, William, 11
jouissance, 143, 166, 169–170, 175–176, 212, 216, 221, 226–228, 230–233, 249, 260, 279
judgment, 146–149, 151–154, 182–183, 216

Klein, Melanie, 23, 41, 255, 285n8; on reparation and adaptation, 38
knowledge, 21, 23, 30–34, 39, 53, 98, 106, 140, 144, 180–183, 188, 207, 223, 250–251, 257–258, 263–265, 267, 279

Lacan, Jacques, 31–32, 43; and analytic treatment, 35, 64–65, 221–223, 228–229, 243, 248–251, 263–266; case histories of, 170–171, 177, 230; and failure of sexual relations, 40; and foreclosure, 196; and transference, 124, 220; and women analysts, 41, 168, 250
Lacan, Jacques, works: "Anxiety (Seminar X)," 167; "The Direction of the Treatment and the Principles of Its Power" (1958), 249; *Encore* (1972–1973), 244–247; *The Knowledge of the Psychoanalyst* (1971–1972), 50–51; "A Lacanian Psychosis" (1980), 95–97; "L'Etourdit" (1972a), 148, 167; *The Logic of Fantasy* (1966–1967), 256 (*see also* Freud, Sigmund, works: "A Child Is Being Beaten"); "Propos sur l'hysterie" (1977), 122; *Television* (1973), 97; "Variations on the Standard Treatment" (1953), 254–256, 266–267 (*see also* psychoanalytic institution; training analysis); "The Youth of Gide, or, The Letter of Desire," 248
law, 37, 136–139, 146, 148, 152, 196–197, 200–201, 225, 241, 248, 251, 258
Leclaire, Serge, 217, 222, 232–235,

limit, 56, 90, 141, 148, 176, 187–190, 208, 211, 226, 241, 248; as border/boundary, 6, 44–45, 48, 77–79, 81, 83, 95–98, 122, 167, 219, 232; confrontation with, 36, 64–66, 92–93, 229
listening, 3–5, 10, 14, 17–18, 20–21, 28, 50, 54–55, 69, 122–124, 134, 148, 154, 169, 194, 216, 226, 246–247, 267, 271
localization, 276–277, 281–282
love, 23, 31, 80, 84, 110- 111, 114, 164, 184, 186, 188, 191, 207, 214, 221, 241–247, 258, 260

madness, 24, 32–33, 98, 181, 190–201, 230, 248, 289n2
marriage, 104–105, 169, 170–171, 209, 213, 260, 268–270; failure of, 108, 113–114, 116, 160–161
masculinity, 62, 111, 113, 160, 168, 175, 204–205, 238; and impotence, 105–107, 158–160, 168, 225; and sexual bondage, 104–105, 115, 169
masturbation, 80, 158–159, 216, 230, 232, 256, 280
materiality, 184, 256, 281; and language, 40, 51, 55, 58, 167, 197, 204, 206–208, 223, 231–232, 264–265; and models, 79–80, 109, 145; and pain, 39, 44, 47
maternal, 19, 53, 59, 108–109, 126, 129, 166, 204–209, 212–213, 220, 225–226, 230, 238, 260, 269–271, 279, 288n3, 289n3. *See also* separation
melancholia, 68, 80, 82–83, 154, 209, 211; and hysteria, 78, 81, 83; and loss of libido, 81–82, 103–104; and melancholic guilt, 114–116, 270 (*see also* guilt); and mourning, 43, 57, 99, 114, 127, 163, 269–272; and psychoanalysis, 151–152, 210–211. *See also* Freud, Sigmund, works: "Mourning and Melancholia"
memory, 9, 69, 73, 84, 94,104–105, 162, 220–221, 232, 240, 250. *See also* Freud, Sigmund, works: "A Disturbance of Memory"; hysteria: hysterical amnesia
metaphor, 53, 165, 168, 173, 177, 181–184, 186, 188, 194, 196–197, 219
metonymy, 99, 173, 204, 218, 225, 280
Miller, Jacques-Alain, 217

music, 72–73, 88, 98–99, 126, 128–129, 141, 145–146, 203. *See also* rhythm
mystic, 11, 19, 85, 112, 145, 190, 208, 287n3
myth, 9, 112, 143, 150, 182, 184, 214, 250, 261–262, 271, 281, 283n2; of Scylla and Charybdis, 257. *See also* group psychology: and collective narrative

Nancy, Jean-Luc: joyful hysteria, 188–190; psychoanalysis of touch, 181, 185, 188, 191–192
narcissism, 103, 106, 181, 184, 224–225, 234, 258–261, 265–266, 289
negation, 31–32, 36–37, 55, 59, 91, 149, 168–169, 192, 217, 229, 241
neurasthenia, 156, 159–161, 168, 288n2
Nietzsche, Friedrich: *On the Genealogy of Morals* (1887), 49; *The Will to Power* (1901), 144
nightmare, 94, 98, 230
nihilism, 80, 116, 139, 250; and pessimism, 158, 160, 176
Nock, A. D., 49–50
nonsense, 3, 28, 120, 124, 197–198
Novalis, 182, 184. *See also* Bachelard, Gaston

object, 43, 53, 70, 89, 110, 115, 128, 133, 152, 163–164, 166–167, 169, 177–178, 181, 217, 220, 233–235, 282; sexual/love, 78–80, 103, 111, 127; lost, 82, 113, 162–164, 212, 223–226, 232–233; research, 137–138; art/aesthetic, 210–211, 214; partial, 140, 164, 209, 229, 267–268; surplus, 174, 176–177, 181, 183, 214; phobic, 207
obsession, 51, 66–68, 70–72, 77, 75, 159, 231, 259
Oedipus, 132, 182, 218, 232, 241, 249, 260, 266, 268
orgasm, 157, 161, 166

pain, 36, 39, 44, 47, 58, 81, 82, 130, 153, 157, 163, 205, 211, 213–214, 217, 229–230, 276, 281
paternal, 93–95, 108–109, 122, 124, 151, 183, 209, 213, 225, 238, 241–242, 256–257, 259–260, 268–269, 280–281
patient, 54–56, 125–130, 130–133, 143, 198, 201, 204, 214, 216, 226, 233, 242, 259, 270–271; relation to analyst, 33–34, 36, 153, 173, 209, 217, 220, 231, 246–247, 255–257, 265, 271 (*see also* training analysis); dreams of, 127–129, 154, 211–213, 225, 229–231, 234
paranoia, 6, 67–68, 75, 123; and philosophy, 112
perversion, 137, 157
phallus, 55, 122–123, 152, 164, 166, 174, 265
philosophy, 5–6, 25–28, 49, 54, 112, 214, 219, 254, 283n2, 289n1; history of, 20, 139; Immanuel Kant, 139–140; and philosophical archaeology, 139–141
pleasure, 14, 22, 31, 80–85, 143, 158, 160–164, 175–177, 187, 191, 210, 223, 226, 231–232, 242–243, 256, 275, 286n1, 287n1. *See also* Freud, Sigmund: pleasure principle
pregnancy, 124–125, 154, 157, 159–160, 205–208, 269–271, 276–279, 281; and abortion, 212; metaphors of, 227
prohibition, 105, 111, 182, 195, 205, 269
projection, 67, 74, 187, 251
psychoanalyst, 2–6, 10, 42–43, 116, 124, 144, 153, 189, 219, 231, 235, 250–251, 262, 266, 284n2; attack on, 16–17, 209; body of, 16–18, 36, 43, 51–52, 54, 59, 115, 144, 265, 272; conversion of, 11, 25, 42, 60, 110, 116, 149, 217, 226–227, 234–235, 243, 254, 263, 267, 272, 284n2; desire of, 7, 15, 43–44, 51, 150, 168, 221–222, 227, 230, 243, 250; forgetting of, 220; role/place of, 148, 171, 204, 209, 216–218, 221, 235, 249, 257–259
psychoanalytic institution, 2, 12, 24–25, 41–42, 83, 152, 168, 192, 195, 244, 248, 266–269, 272; history of, 93, 95, 100, 118, 122–123, 142, 193, 229, 242, 254–255, 265 (*see also* Lacan, Jacques: "Variations on the Standard Treatment"); and professionalization, 130–131, 243, 255. *See also* training analysis
psychoanalytic treatment, 34, 37, 42, 46, 116, 124, 134, 143–144, 148, 177, 190, 201, 206–208, 213–214, 228, 231, 233–235, 250, 255, 264–267; architecture of, 45; contemporary relevance of, 45, 227, 269; as embodiment, 15, 50–51 53–55, 56, 59, 181, 185, 188, 192, 205, 223; and hypnosis, 110–111, 184

psychosis, 85, 95–98, 114, 123, 193–194, 196, 284n3, 286n1, 290n2

real, 94–95, 107–108, 113, 149, 153, 196, 232, 256
redemption, 136–139, 141, 227–228, 259–260
religion, 2, 5–6, 11, 25, 49–50, 112, 136–138, 141, 186, 211, 214, 227–228; and Christianity, 49, 177, 191, 208, 278; and theology, 46, 136, 142, 217
religious conversion, 39, 46, 49–50, 90, 112, 136–138, 147, 177, 208, 227–228
repetition, 52–54, 107, 131–132, 143–144, 161, 208, 217–219, 223–226, 230–233, 238–239, 242, 244, 270
repression, 68–71, 76, 82, 141, 143, 161–163, 196, 220, 232, 251, 256
resistance, 54, 63, 69, 143, 199, 201; overcoming, 104–105; and the psychoanalyst, 144; to the sexual, 110, 188
revelation, 17, 33–36, 59, 140, 142, 147, 193, 213, 233–234, 250, 259, 263, 265
rhythm, 3, 5, 48, 59, 66, 69, 75, 170, 177, 190, 217, 227, 231
ritual, 6, 35–36, 105, 194, 196, 209–211, 214, 275

sadism, 2, 105, 108, 231, 248, 280
scotomization, 70–73, 113, 220
sense, 31, 152–153, 180–181, 185–191, 194, 197, 200
self-analysis, 26, 28, 182, 195, 213–214, 220, 225, 234, 238–239, 254, 261, 267–269, 272, 286n1; and self-eclipsing, 228–229; and self-preservation, 209, 212; and self-satisfaction, 216, 241
separation, 21, 90–91, 98–99, 127, 134, 147, 152, 162–168, 171, 173–174, 186, 191, 208, 214, 246, 276, 282
sexuality, 22, 39, 51, 59, 63, 76–77, 82–84, 110–111, 114, 127, 152, 162, 167, 184, 278; and alienation, 21–22, 157–159, 212, 272; asexuality, 102, 104 111, 198; bisexuality, 285n5; diphasic, 111, 208; homosexuality, 112, 123, 278–279, 285n7; and sexual fantasy, 184; and sexual intercourse, 104–109, 116, 156, 158–159, 169, 207, 226–227; and sexual love, 109–111, 114–115, 221 (*see also* love; object: sexual/love); and sexual research, 21, 153, 205, 278; and sexual satisfaction, 107, 110, 114, 143, 158, 160, 212, 216, 223, 226–228, 262. See also Freud, Sigmund, works: *Three Essays on the Theory of Sexuality*
Shakespeare, William: *Hamlet*, 218–219, 254; *King Lear*, 241–242
signifier, 51–52, 100, 158, 187, 190, 198, 200, 232, 225, 234, 250–251, 282; and language, 121–122, 141–142, 149, 181, 194–200, 204, 216, 223, 289n2; and signifying chain/system, 74, 196–197, 221, 256–261
silence, 36, 121, 155, 188, 197, 204, 208, 215, 259, 265
sovereign, 137–138, 142. See also Agamben, Giorgio: political theology
spiritual, 11, 177, 181, 186, 190
splitting, 45, 66, 73, 84, 111, 139–140, 182, 207–208, 210, 214, 220, 227, 264, 268; and partial measures, 158, 160, 241, 262; of speech, 256–257
sublimation, 85, 114–115, 143, 157, 230, 233, 243, 262
superego, 36, 42–43, 47, 127, 137, 152–153, 161, 164, 191, 234, 241, 255, 266; and femininity, 38–39; and injunction, 82–83, 88, 190–191, 205, 210, 214, 233, 260
symbol, 73–74, 109, 142, 164, 196, 244, 256. See also body: and mnemic symbol
symptom, 34, 65–66, 68–71, 74, 76, 80, 84, 94, 103, 109, 112, 127, 143, 188, 190, 204, 207–208, 251, 264, 277, 281–282; *belle indifference* of, 162; and objectlessness, 163, 191

temporality: disordering/splintering of, 35, 52, 54, 69, 74–75, 90, 93, 133, 208, 251; and history, 140–141, 217; and horoscopes/dates, 88–90, 99–100; and sexuality, 141, 158–159, 208
tension, 67, 80–81, 142–144, 162, 187, 192, 210, 232, 266
topology, 97, 113, 115, 144, 187, 208, 216, 224, 225, 277, 281; and folding, 31, 74, 186, 189,

197, 199, 210, 228; and psychoanalytic models, 78, 144, 161–162, 223–224, 255
training analysis, 242, 250, 254, 261, 266–268; and conversion of patient to analyst, 41–42, 44, 53, 221–223, 227, 234, 254–255; and desire to become an analyst, 43, 266–267
transference, 51, 65, 74, 77, 116, 144, 151, 153, 170–174, 220–222, 230, 242, 271
trauma, 46, 74, 130, 136–137, 141, 147, 161–162, 206, 208, 212–214; and psychoanalysis, 51–52, 226, 260, 269; transmissions of, 39, 150
tumescence, 21, 166, 168, 170–171

uncanny, 56, 105, 129, 209, 261–262, 270
unconscious, 66, 75–76, 118, 134, 138, 145, 150, 165, 187, 221, 227–228, 242–244, 249, 256, 259, 265, 267

violence, 45–46, 116, 120, 128, 131–132, 166, 201, 229–230, 232; and aggression, 38–39, 161, 226, 231, 267, 285n1, 285n8; and violation, 220. *See also* death drive; wound
virtual, 25, 33, 88, 173–174
voice, 148–150, 152–153, 164, 182, 228

waiting, 35–36, 71–72, 84, 123
wound, 23, 38, 58, 91–93, 98, 212, 217, 224, 229, 244, 281; and wish, 95, 230, 244, 264, 285n6
writing, 21, 57–58, 84, 104, 109, 115, 118, 172, 177, 189, 200, 214, 219, 228, 235, 248, 276; and bodily exscription/inscription, 186, 190, 200–201, 211, 213, 217, 220, 233, 260, 282; a letter, 89–91, 95, 124, 213, 278; and name/signature, 212, 261–262, 270–272, 280–281; scene of, 30, 33, 238; and transmission of psychoanalysis, 254, 265

GPSR Authorized Representative: Easy Access System Europe, Mustamäe tee 50, 10621 Tallinn, Estonia, gpsr.requests@easproject.com